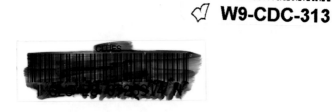
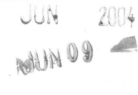

How Children Learn to Be Healthy

The goal of this book is to explore the ways in which health behavior develops in childhood in the context of childhood socialization processes. The book reviews the historical and contemporary perspectives utilized in portraying the dynamics of children's physical health. It provides a developmental analysis of children's and parents' attitudes and behavior concerning children's health; assesses the role of parents, schools, and the media in influencing children's health attitudes and behavior; and examines how health attitudes, behaviors, and outcomes are affected by the social ecology of children's rearing environments.

Barbara J. Tinsley is Professor of Psychology and Chair of the Program in Human Development at the University of California, Riverside.

INTERNATIONAL STUDIES ON CHILD
AND ADOLESCENT HEALTH

Steering Committee:

Klaus Hurrelmann, *University of Bielefeld, Germany*
Candace Currie, *University of Edinburgh, United Kingdom*
Vivian B. Rasmussen, *WHO Regional Office for Europe,*
  Copenhagen, Denmark

The series ISCAH aims at publishing books on the health and disease status of children, adolescents, and young adults and on intervention strategies in medicine, psychology, sociology, public health, and political science. The series is supported by the international research network Health Behavior in School Children (HBSC) and is sponsored by the World Health Organization (WHO) Regional Office for Europe.

In this series:

Diabetic Adolescents and Their Families, Inge Seiffge-Krenke
How Children Learn to Be Healthy, Barbara J. Tinsley

How Children Learn to Be Healthy

Barbara J. Tinsley
University of California, Riverside

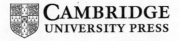

CAMBRIDGE
UNIVERSITY PRESS

PUBLISHED BY THE PRESS SYNDICATE OF THE UNIVERSITY OF CAMBRIDGE
The Pitt Building, Trumpington Street, Cambridge, United Kingdom

CAMBRIDGE UNIVERSITY PRESS
The Edinburgh Building, Cambridge CB2 2RU, UK
40 West 20th Street, New York, NY 10011-4211, USA
477 Williamstown Road, Port Melbourne, VIC 3207, Australia
Ruiz de Alarcón 13, 28014 Madrid, Spain
Dock House, The Waterfront, Cape Town 8001, South Africa

http://www.cambridge.org

First published 2003

Printed in the United Kingdom at the University Press, Cambridge

Typeface Times Ten 10/13 pt.   *System* LATEX 2_ε [TB]

A catalog record for this book is available from the British Library.

Library of Congress Cataloging in Publication Data
Tinsley, Barbara J., 1950–
How children learn to be healthy / Barbara J. Tinsley.
   p.   cm. – (International studies on child and adolescent health)
Includes bibliographical references and index.
ISBN 0-521-58098-6 – ISBN 0-521-52418-0 (pbk.)
1. Health behavior in children.   2. Health behavior.   3. Medicine, Preventive.
4. Health promotion.   I. Title.   II. Series.
RA776.9 .T54   2002
613′.0432 – dc21   2002022289

ISBN 0 521 58098 6 hardback
ISBN 0 521 52418 0 paperback

For my parents, Belle Margaret Rozalsky and Irving Rozalsky

Contents

Acknowledgments

My first thanks go to the thousands of women, men, and children who have shared their stories, beliefs, and perspectives about health, wellness, and illness with me throughout my career. Their willingness to talk about their experiences and teach me about their lives has made this book possible.

The National Institutes of Child and Human Development provided funding for several of the studies this book draws upon, and I am grateful for the support I received from them to conduct this research.

I would also like to thank Julia Hough, my commissioning editor at Cambridge University Press, for her unwavering patience with me as I wrote this book over several years. Additionally, I am very grateful to Helen Wheeler, my production editor at Cambridge University Press, for coordinating all the tasks at the Press necessary to complete this book, and to Helen Greenberg, the copy editor of this book, who carefully edited the manuscript.

Many thanks are due to my current and former graduate, undergraduate, and medical students, who have been my research partners in these studies. Conducting research with them has been a creative, stimulating, and enjoyable process, and my students have been a continuing source of learning and inspiration for me over the years.

I have been fortunate to live my life filled with many bright, spirited, and creative minds. And more fortunate still that many of these wonderful minds and hearts have been generous with their intelligence, time, support, and viewpoints. In particular, I am deeply grateful and appreciative to Ross D. Parke, my former husband and current colleague, without whose wisdom, scholarship, confidence, intellect, humor, and photographic mind for references this book would never have come to fruition. His constant admonitions to "go the high road" and "move it up a level" have been invaluable in the writing of this book (despite my limited ability to appreciate them at the time!).

I also thank my other colleagues in the Department of Psychology at the University of California, Riverside, and in particular, my Chair, John Ashe, for unwavering support and confidence in my past, present, and future endeavors.

I owe very special thanks to the many physicians who have given me generous amounts of their understanding of and experience with their patients and their families. In particular, two of the physicians with whom I have worked stand out in this regard. One is Dr. Gary Feinberg, an otorhinolaryngologist, who graciously allowed me to spend a 6-month sabbatical leave traipsing along next to him, observing surgeries, office visits, and hospital visits. His effective and compassionate manner with his patients was stimulating and encouraging, and I learned from him about the power of empathy and skill in healing. The second is Dr. Alan Kwasman, the best pediatrician in the world. He treats his "moms" with respect and caring and his child patients with humor and devotion. Having had the opportunity to observe him with his patients and their families in his pediatric practice for more than a decade has been the finest education one could have in the art and science of medicine. My professional association and friendship with him have been a treasured privilege in my "gifted life." The children who receive his care are very fortunate indeed, and more than anyone I know, he has made a real difference in the lives of children and their families.

I am unreservedly grateful for and awed by the love and faith of my children, Sarah Villareal, Jennifer Tinsley, and Zachary Parke, and my son-in-law, Jose Manuel Villareal. Each, in his or her own way, has taught me everything about being a mother that cannot be said in a book. They are the treasures of my life, and I will always be eternally and infinitely grateful to them for sharing with me, loving me, and letting me love them. Living with and loving my stepchildren, Gillian Parke, Timothy Parke, and Megan Parke, has also been a privilege, and I wholeheartedly thank them for their trust, friendship, and love. My sisters, Susan Rozalsky and Laura Rozalsky, have known me longer than anyone else on earth, and my relationships with them have been rich, deep, and the most interesting of any in my life. I am grateful for their support, love, and friendship over the years of our lives. Rose Sadowsky, my aunt, has been a life-long inspiration for me. She is one of the most educated and intelligent people I have known, and she has always believed in me ... a very powerful combination.

I also thank Rosa Stopnicki, who continues to teach me about mothering, the healing properties of chicken soup, and all other parts of life. I will never cease to be grateful for her wisdom, intuition, and kindness. I am also grateful to Elan Stopnitzky for his friendship and trust, and for all the other children in my life and outside my life, who deserve to live a life of health and wellness.

Finally, there is my life partner, Ben Zion (Benny) Stopnitzky. Throughout many of the months of writing and revising this book, his love, intellect, good heart, and scrambled eggs sustained and invigorated me. With his presence in my life, I have learned to think and solve problems in more logical ways. His insistent challenge to me to grow and change has resulted in many new perspectives on old issues. And most of all, I thank him for his wonderful sense of humor and amazing ability to make me laugh. Benny's support and caring have become the foundation of my personal, spiritual, and professional lives and, if I am very lucky, will continue to do so for the remainder of my life.

How Children Learn to Be Healthy

Introduction

The goal of this book is to explore the ways in which health behavior develops in childhood in the context of childhood socialization processes. In the first chapter, several issues are presented. The first aim is to define the state of children's health in the United States. Most parents want their children to be safe and healthy, but implementing that desire can be a difficult and challenging process. According to recent surveys of Americans' health habits, American parents and children are fatter, more stressed out, exercise less, and pay less attention to what they eat than ever before. Many of the most serious health and social problems facing our nation today have their origins and potential solutions in health behaviors developed in childhood. At least 8 out of 10 of the leading causes of death – heart disease, cancer, strokes, injuries, chronic lung disease, diabetes, liver disease, and atherosclerosis – are strongly related to such behaviors and conditions as diet and obesity, exercise, smoking, and drinking alcohol. What must be addressed is that these health behaviors begin in childhood. By the age of 12, more than 40% of American children have at least one modifiable risk factor for coronary heart disease (Richter et al., 2000).

Physicians and other public health and medical professionals now know enough about how to keep children well so that debilitating illness and disease should be much less frequent than they are in the United States. Yet, in this country, children's health suffers from birth. The overall U.S. infant mortality rate ranks 22nd worldwide; 9 out of every 1,000 children in the United States die before age 1, which is twice the infant mortality rate of Japan. Between 30% and 55% of 2-year-old American children are not adequately immunized, and the percentages of underimmunized children are much higher in major U.S. cities. Today, a 2-year-old in

Mexico City is more likely to be fully immunized than a similar child in the United States. Even many older children are not staying healthy in the United States. Although many parents say that they try to limit the salt, caffeine, fat, and sugar in their children's diets, many children have very unhealthy diets. Only about one-third of children always wear helmets and other protective gear when riding bicycles, skates, or skateboards, and over two-thirds wear them only sometimes. Several recent studies have demonstrated important gaps in the fitness levels of children, and measured declines in physical activity over the past decade have been documented. Nearly one-third of children aged 3 to 17 are overweight for their age and gender.

In an effort to understand the etiology of children's health status, this chapter has, as its second goal, to review the historical and contemporary perspectives utilized in portraying the dynamics of child health. Until recently, the dominant model of children's health has been biomedical, simultaneously emphasizing biological models of wellness and illness and disregarding social, psychological, and behavioral dimensions of health. However, the dominance of the strict biomedical model of disease is lessening, and a model incorporating concern with behavior and the whole person is much more prevalent in current health research and clinical settings. Developmental models have also undergone a series of revisions over the past three decades, resulting in increased recognition of biological conditions such as wellness and illness as factors in development. Not only are genetic and constitutionally based differences among infants and children more often acknowledged as having an important impact on health and development, but the continuing importance of biological factors, such as adequate nutrition for proper cognitive development, is increasingly addressed. New developmental models that incorporate both biological and experiential components have appeared. These models demonstrate that neither biological nor experiential factors alone yield adequate understanding of development and that only by combining these components can one better understand development. With the development of these new medical and developmental models has come increasing interest on the part of those concerned with children's health in the contribution of an expanded range of variables to child health. The effects of such factors as children's health attitudes, knowledge, and behavior, as well as the influence of children's socialization agents and environments on child health status, are increasingly recognized as critical to wellness promotion and illness prevention in childhood. Moreover, the developmental progression of these children's health orientations is being increasingly recognized as a critical issue in efforts to promote children's health. The final aim of this chapter is to frame several important questions that are addressed in the remainder of the book, including how children's developmental status relates to their health orientation and the socialization of that orientation, and what familial or other social environmental conditions provide the opportunity for and promote the acquisition of children's health knowledge, attitudes, and behavior.

Chapter 2 presents a thorough and detailed developmental analysis of children's attitudes toward an understanding of health concepts. Children's developmental ideas about these concepts, as exemplified by the classic work of Rashkis (1965), Bibace and Walsh (1980), Campbell (1975), Natapoff (1978), Perrin and Gerrity (1981), and Simeonsson, Buckley, and Monson (1979), are considered in this chapter. Children's stage-related understanding of specific health concepts, such as contagion and germs, are also presented in this chapter, as researched by Wilkinson (1988), Nagy (1951, 1953), Siegal (Siegal & Peterson, 1999), and others. Controversy concerning the timing and sophistication with which children achieve these understandings is also explored and explained. Alternative cognitive explanatory models for children's health understanding are also portrayed, including script theory as developed by Nelson (1986) and children's intuitive theories of behavior as described by Carey (1985).

A second focus of the research on children's health attitudes and behavior is individual differences in these areas, as reflected in such constructs as health locus of control, perceived vulnerability to health problems, and health motivation in work by such researchers as Gochman (1987), Parcel and Meyer (1978), and others. A following section suggests an integration of the stage theory and individual differences perspectives on children's health understanding. The role of health attitudes in children's preventive health behavior, and its relations to children's developmental status, is also explored in this chapter. The moderate relations between children's health-related attitudes and health behavior are discussed, and theoretical reasons for this modest link are offered. Finally, children's health behavior is described. A developmental portrait of children's self-initiated health behavior is offered, including nutrition, exercise, and other health and safety domains. While most of young children's preventive health care is initiated and managed by parents, children become, with age, increasingly able and expected to manage their own preventive health. The chapter ends with descriptions of a unique context in children's health behavior: their self-initiated visits to health care providers in school such as school nurses.

Parents' influence on their children's health through a variety of mechanisms, including their beliefs and behavior, is considered in Chapter 3. This chapter examines the developmental progression of how parents' beliefs affect children's health attitudes, behavior, and outcomes. While parents' health attitudes are a somewhat indirect influence on children's preventive health behavior, they usually function via their influence on parents' behavior rather than by direct communication to the child, and the dynamics of this influence change as the child develops. Developmental research investigating such aspects as the value parents place on health, parents' perceptions of the seriousness of and susceptibility to disease, parents' attitudes toward medication, the seriousness with which parents consider their children's symptom-reporting, and parental health locus of control is presented in this chapter. An important distinction is made between parents' beliefs about their own health and parents' beliefs about their children's health, and the relative predictive value of each in determining how parents will act on behalf of their children's health. Family- and culturally based belief systems that affect parents' health attitudes are also discussed. The impact of parent health-related beliefs on child health behavior and outcomes over the course of child development is also presented. The mechanisms by which parents' beliefs about children's health influence child health behavior and outcomes are outlined, including a discussion of children's developmental status and parents' thought processes that intervene to mediate parents' health socialization strategies and children's outcomes. The conceptual framework is guided by recent social information processing models as applied to parental health beliefs and decision making.

Parental childrearing behavior, in the context of children's developmental status, is explored in Chapters 4 and 5 as pathways through which parents' beliefs influence children's health. The work of such investigators as Pratt (1973) and Lau and Klepper (1988), and cross-cultural work by Olvera-Ezzell, Power, and Cousins (1990) and Yamasaki (1995) on the impact of non-health-specific parental child-rearing behavior on children's health behavior, are utilized to illustrate this path. Other mechanisms of childhood socialization of health behavior by parents, such as modeling and reinforcement, and establishment and enforcement of child health behavior, are discussed theoretically and empirically in great detail. Moving beyond the individual level of analysis to a consideration of the family as a health socialization unit is explored as a useful framework for further understanding the dynamics of childhood health learning. With this perspective, three important but somewhat neglected aspects of parents' influence on child health are examined with respect to child development: the impact of parent–child emotional interactions on children's health, the effect of parents' interactions with others (e.g., marital interaction), and the impact of parents' own health on children's health. A neo-Vygotskian perspective is offered as a way of conceptualizing the socialization strategies of parents in relation to the promotion of children's health.

As children develop, peers and schools play increasingly important roles in determining their health attitudes and behavior, and their influence is examined in Chapter 6. Peers provide either complementary or competing sources of health influence, along with parents and other socializing agents. Research on childhood peer socialization in health contexts, as a function of child developmental status, is reviewed. The theoretical and empirical work on the changing relations between parental control and peer influence as children develop is applied to health contexts, as exemplified by work by Steinberg, Lamborn, Dornbusch, and Darling (1992), Smetana, Kochanska, and Chuang (2000), and others. Schools have been demonstrated to significantly influence children's behavior, apart from the family. Effective school-based health education teaches children what healthful and unhealthful behaviors are and the consequences of practicing these behaviors. Moreover, in schools, interventions designed to modify children's health attitudes and behaviors are most often initiated. The advantages of school-based health education are presented, together with a developmental analysis of formal school-based education efforts and their efficacy. Deficits in current school-based health education are examined, and its potential importance is evaluated.

Parents, schools, and peers are not the only influences on children's health; television viewing and exposure to other media, examined in Chapter 7, help shape children's health attitudes and behavior. In light of statistics documenting the amount of time children spend watching television, which includes a surprising number and variety of events that have clear implications for health and risk, this chapter analyzes in detail research on television's influence on children's health. Developmental aspects of how children learn about health from television are presented. Then the content of television is examined; commercials are particularly salient sources of influence on children's health, with billions of dollars spent each year by corporations to televise commercial advertisements for nonnutritional foods, alcohol, and tobacco products, which are attractive to children and detrimental to their health. Other television programming, including soap operas, televised movies, MTV videos, and prime-time presentations, are also examined for their messages and impact on children's health attitudes and behavior. The effects of children's television viewing on several aspects of health beliefs and behavior are then examined, including the impact of programs depicting suicide, food intake, medicine-taking, sexuality, and standards of beauty and attractiveness. Finally, the indirect impact of television watching on children's health is explored, which concerns how television alters time use and activity choice in children. The consequences for children's health of reduced recreational physical activity when television is available are presented.

In Chapter 8, the ways in which children's health attitudes, behavior, and health status are affected in yet another way, namely, by the social ecology in which children and families are located (cf. Bronfenbrenner, 2000), are discussed. This ecology promotes or constrains child health behavior and outcomes. Although demographic status, specifically socioeconomic status, has traditionally been the focus of efforts to describe and predict children's health, in this chapter it is suggested that social class is not an explanatory variable with respect to health. In most cases, social class merely describes parents and children who vary in health attitudes, behavior, and actual health. Parents and children of higher social class usually experience better health services access and utilization, as well as better health. Although the mechanisms by which social class affects health are poorly understood, parental socioeconomic variables such as education, occupation, and income are clearly associated with children's health status. These factors also strongly influence aspects of the health environment in which children develop, including such aspects as parent–child interaction, parental beliefs and attitudes, physical environment attributes (e.g., space, crowding, cleanliness, noise), organization, regularity and predictability of schedules and caregiving, and the availability of food, materials, and other resources. The research of several investigators exploring the relation between health and environment in childhood within a developmental perspective is presented. The developmental trajectories of how poor environments compromise children's health are also explored in this chapter.

1

Mechanisms and Consequences of Socializing Children to Be Healthy

Heart disease and cancer are the first and second leading causes of death in the United States. Although great strides have been made in reducing deaths from heart disease in the past 20 years, due to improvements in treatment for hypertension and myocardial infarction and changes in diet, smoking levels, and exercise patterns, deaths from many cancers continue to increase. Cigarette smoking is the leading cause of lung cancer in both men and women. We know that 80% of smokers begin to smoke during adolescence and that attitudes learned in childhood and adolescence are the most powerful predictors of smoking in adulthood. Imagine how much additional reduction in the number of deaths caused by these two major killers could be achieved if children began to eat healthy diets in childhood, if they never started to smoke cigarettes, and if physical exercise was a natural part of every child's life.

There appears to be an inadequate U.S. national commitment to prevention and health promotion; our national investment in prevention is estimated at less than 5% of the total annual health cost (Stone et al., 2000), and without this orientation toward prevention, the prospects for children's health and functioning cannot be improved. Money is available to provide expensive hospital care for those with serious illnesses; thousands of preterm and otherwise sick infants are hospitalized for months at a time. But Americans make inadequate attempts to improve children's lives before they get sick, and many of today's children will reach adulthood unhealthy.

In order to understand the etiology of children's health status, it is important to review the historical and contemporary perspectives utilized in portraying the dynamics of child health. Until recently, the dominant model of children's health has been biomedical, simultaneously emphasizing biological models of wellness and illness and disregarding social, psychological, and behavioral dimensions of health (Engel, 1977; Tinsley & Parke, 1984). However, the dominance of the strict biomedical model of disease is lessening, and a model incorporating concern with behavior and the whole person is much more prevalent in health research, in both academic and clinical settings.

Sameroff's (1989) transactional model of development suggests that two continua – a continuum of reproductive causality, which includes both genetic constitutional factors and birth-related trauma, and a continuum of caretaking causality, which includes the social, intellectual, and physical environments – are necessary for adequate prediction of developmental outcomes. Other models such as systems theory approaches similarly stress the necessity of considering the complex interplay between biological and experiential factors (Ramey, MacPhee, & Yeates, 1982; see also Sameroff, 1982). These shifts suggest that the traditional medical and developmental models have undergone modification, resulting in mutual movement to incorporate major tenets of each.

Other factors have also contributed to the emerging redefinition of the relation between traditional medical and developmental models of child health and development. Due to a decrease in child mortality and morbidity rates (brought about by the conquest of a number of major infectious diseases by biological medical science), pediatric medical science is also preoccupied with two major concerns: (1) the prevention of chronic diseases related to lifestyle and social environment later in life and (2) parents' requests for child-rearing advice (Doherty & Campbell, 1988; Tinsley & Parke, 1984).

Currently, medical science is significantly focused on illnesses caused by noninfectious processes (e.g., heart disease, cancer). Single microbiologic factors are not solely responsible for these types of diseases; lifestyle factors such as diet and smoking are considered to be significant contributors. Preventive measures, emphasizing lifestyle and behavior, are highly valued ways in which to maximize wellness. Health professionals increasingly target many of their efforts to influence children's lifestyle and behavior in the belief that health habits are formed early and persist throughout life. Considerable work has been accomplished utilizing a variety of methodologies and paradigms, which illustrate the importance of such nonbiological factors for children's health.

Secondly, parents' requests for childrearing advice are taking increasing amounts of pediatricians' professional time. Estimates of the extent to which pediatric primary care visits involve childrearing, behavior problems, or other psychological components vary from 37% to 50% (Duff, Rowe, & Anderson, 1973; Glascoe, 1999). Thus, pediatric medical professionals spend far less time ameliorating illnesses caused by infection and more time helping parents and children to shape health and other types of child behavior.

In summary, on the pediatric side, the traditional and formerly dominant medical model of disease, which conceptualizes disease as a deviation from normative biological functioning, is being replaced by medical models that address social, psychological, and behavioral dimensions of disease (Engel, 1977; Tinsley & Parke, 1984). In addition, developmentalists' past concentration on behavioral models that give little explicit recognition to biological factors is diminishing. Practitioners in the fields of both pediatrics and child psychology demonstrate concern with the effects on health and development of psychosocial and behavioral factors.

With the development of this new interest on the part of medical professionals in children's health attitudes and behavior, and of social scientists in child health, has come a substantial increase in research on children's health attitudes and behavior. For those who are interested in the factors influencing children's health (e.g., for preventive or ameliorative purposes), this emerging model will be useful for specifying nonbiological correlates and causes of children's wellness and illness.

Mechanisms

The mechanisms of children's health-related attitudes, and of behavior acquisition and socialization, have been the focus of theoretical and empirical attention. Two issues have been explored. First, what familial or other social environmental conditions provide the opportunity for the acquisition of attitudes or behaviors that are necessary for child wellness? Second, what are the mechanisms that facilitate the acquisition and socialization of these attitudes and behaviors? As will be presented in this book, the research, to date has focused on several possible factors that may be involved in explaining childhood health socialization. In studies of child health attitudes and behavior, the explanatory burden has fallen on three categories of variables: (1) the child's background and characteristics (i.e., developmental status, demographics, personality variables, and possibly gender), (2) extrafamilial agents (peers, schools, media), and (3) the parents' and family's relational and interaction variables.

The most common and well-researched way in which children learn about health is through familial relations. The research suggests that parents and families provide models of health attitudes and behavior, demonstrating, teaching, and reinforcing specific health attitudes and behavior, as influenced by background characteristics such as demographics and parents' personality variables (Garralda, 2000). Children are hypothesized to learn concepts of health and health skills as a result of repeated opportunities for practice of these behaviors in the home. Evidence suggests that these concepts and skills are utilized by children, as they get older, in other health behavior–eliciting situations, such as with friends and in school. Exposure to these alternative contexts serves to modify these health attitudes and behaviors. Nevertheless, the research indicates that children's health attitudes and behaviors appear to be more similar than dissimilar to those of their parents (Wiehl & Tinsley, 1999).

2

Children's Health Understanding and Behavior

Children's Understanding of Health

Children's understanding of and attitudes toward health are usually conceptualized in one of two ways. The first is a focus on children's understanding of health-related concepts, including the causes of illness, health knowledge, and other related issues. These can be characterized as reflecting the cognitive-structural tradition, as exemplified by Piaget. This work focuses on age-related normative changes in children's attitudes and ideas. The second perspective considers children's health attitudes and behavior from an individual differences perspective.

Children's Understanding of Health-Related Concepts: Stage Theory

With respect to children's attitudes about health, several domains have been the subject of investigation. These include children's ideas, knowledge, and understanding of health and illness. Gellert (1962) found developmental trends in children's understanding of how their bodies work, with children 9 years of age and older able to describe body systems and their permanence.

Several investigations have been focused on children's developmental ideas about health and illness. Rashkis (1965), in a sample of hospitalized 4- to 8-year-olds, found that the older children were more likely to equate being well with positive attributions than were the younger children. Moreover, all of these children, but especially the older group, believed that physicians, not their parents, were to be held responsible for their health status. The usefulness of this study is limited, however, because the children were hospitalized during the interviews.

Other studies have utilized Piagetian concepts in order to analyze children's systematic understanding of health and illness. In general, these studies suggest that children in the preoperational stage of cognition have ideas about health and illness that are characterized by confusion of cause and effect, superstition, and lack of differentiation (Bibace & Walsh, 1980; Campbell, 1975; Natapoff, 1978; Perrin & Gerrity, 1981; Simeonsson et al., 1979; Walsh & Bibace, 1991). As children reach the concrete operational mode of cognition, their principles of health and illness begin to resemble those of adults, although fairly simplistically. For example, children at this stage have been found to believe that germs cause all illnesses or that wellness depends on conformity to specific rules (Bibace & Walsh, 1980; Perrin & Gerrity, 1981). In the formal operational period, more sophisticated concepts such as infection and preventive health behavior are understandable (Simeonsson et al., 1979).

Developmental Approaches to Children's Understanding of Germs and Contagion

One special focus of investigators interested in children's stage-related understanding of health concepts has been on children's explanations of contagion and germs. In an extensive interview study of children's understanding of germs, Wilkinson (1988) reports age patterns in children's concepts of contagion. Preschool children, according to Wilkinson, are confused about germs because the word *bug* is often used by older children and adults as a synonym for *germ*. Another source of confusion about germs for very young children is their invisibility, in contrast to their powerful ability to cause greatly salient discomfort and dysfunction. Wilkinson found that even preschool children understand that proximity to sick people increases the risk of "catching" an illness. Children of this age reported that germs are able to enter the body through the mouth, through contaminated food, via contact with dirty hands, or by kissing. However, they did not connect their parents' socialization of social routines associated with cleanliness (e.g., washing hands before eating) with parents' attempts to prevent germ contagion. Only by age 7 (consistent with the onset of Piaget's stage of concrete operations) were children able to make sense of the multiple words used for germ analogies. Furthermore, children of this age had a germ classification system that included good germs and bad germs (which cause illness), and they expanded the preschool notion of contagion only through the mouth to include breathing germ-laden air from a sick person. Finally, by adolescence (Piaget's stage of formal operations), children were no longer dependent on such analogies as insects for their understanding of contagion. Moreover, they appeared to have a well-developed understanding of ways to prevent the spread of germs and have internalized responsibility for engaging in behaviors that represent barriers to contagion.

Other researchers studying children's developmental concepts of germs and contagion do not find children as advanced as Wilkinson's study indicates. For example, Nagy, in several early studies (1951, 1953), developmentally assessed children's attitudes about the causes of illness. The results of these studies indicated that it is only children 6 years of age and older who are cognitively capable of understanding concepts associated with infection. However, children between the ages of 6 and 10 believe, according to Nagy, that a single germ causes all kinds of illness; only at age 11 are children starting to understand that specific germs cause specific diseases.

Bibace and Walsh (1980) offer further evidence of concordance between Piagetian states of cognitive development and children's explanations of illness. According to these researchers, preschool children (aged 2–6 years) explain illness phenomenologically, attributing illness to trees, the sun, or magic. Older children (7–10 years of age) understand contamination but can explain how germs cause body illness only vaguely. By age 11, Bibace and Walsh believe that children are capable of fairly sophisticated physiological and psychophysiological explanations of illness. Similarly, Perrin and Gerrity (1981) report data from children 5–13 years of age that suggest a similar cognitive stage analysis of children's understanding of the causes of illness. Specifically, the youngest children believed that illness is magical or a punishment for misbehavior. The middle age group of children in this sample believed that the presence of germs in the body causes illness. Only the oldest children were able to understand the complexity of illness and its multiple causes. This type of study was also conducted by Rozin and his associates (Rozin, Fallon, & Augustoni-Ziskind, 1985). These investigators asked young children to drink glasses of juice that contained such items as used combs and insects. Many children aged 4–6 years drank the juice, demonstrating, according to these researchers, their inability to understand contagion.

How do we reconcile these discrepancies in researchers' estimates of the age at which children become cognitively sophisticated about contagion and illness? Wilkinson (1988) and Siegal (1991) believe that studies demonstrating later understanding of these concepts underestimate children's ability to process these facts due to inadequate research methods. Specifically, they maintain that inadequate attention to the development of a trusting relationship between the interviewers and the child subjects in such studies inhibited the children's ability to communicate their far greater true understanding of the relations between contagion and illness.

States Siegal, "evidence [that young children do not understand contagion and contamination as causes of illness] has often come from studies in which children have been subjected to forms of prolonged or unconventional questioning that may be perceived (by the children) to depart from the conversational rule to be sincere. Under this procedure, children's inconsistent responses . . . may not reflect the depth of their understanding. Rather than lacking knowledge of the causes of illness, they may simply have misinterpreted what they were required to do. For example, children may know that a drink which has been in contact with a foreign object can be harmful and they may reject the object as food. At the same time, they may not be aware that a grown-up might offer children a contaminated drink and insincerely imply . . . that the drink is safe in a well-meaning effort to test their understanding" (1991, pp. 52–53). In a series of four experiments, Siegal (1991) reexamined children's knowledge of contagion and contamination by asking children to evaluate others' explanations for illness, to indicate the likelihood that illness would occur, and to predict their own preventive health behavior. Results of these studies demonstrated, consonant with Wilkinson's (1988) findings, that even very young children understand the association between contagion, contamination, and illness. Siegal attributes his findings of precocity in children's understanding of these relations to his use of "child-friendly" interviewing techniques that incorporate questioning that abides "by rules of conversation and conveys elements of sincerity, non-redundancy, relevance, and clarity" (p. 61).

Finally, and perhaps most interesting, is that several studies find that children's understanding of contagion and illness chronologically parallels children's stages of moral development better than their cognitive understanding of physical causality (Bibace & Walsh, 1980; Perrin & Gerrity, 1981). For example, Kister and Patterson (1980) found an inverse relation between children's understanding of germs and contagion, as a cause of illness, and their belief in immanent justice. Specifically, the results of this study demonstrated that children approximately between the ages of 5 and 10 offer immanent justice explanations (i.e., the belief that inanimate objects can cause natural justice events, or, in other words, that sickness is caused by being naughty) for illness more often than for bad luck or unintentional injuries. Older children, with better concepts of germs and contagion, offer fewer immanent justice explanations for illness than children aged 5 through 10 years. However, Siegal (1991) reminds us that many adults as well as children offer superstitious or magical reasons for natural events such as illness, consistent with immanent justice explanations of illness, and that such magical thinking may be universally present in normal adults (Frazer, 1959; Nemeroff, 1995; Rozin, Markwith, & McCauley, 1994).

Further Evidence of Children's Stage-Related Concepts of Health

Other examples of studies utilizing Piagetian constructs underscore these conclusions. Natapoff (1978), who indicates that children's ideas about health and illness move developmentally from thought characterized by preoperational strategies to concrete operations, studied first, fourth, and seventh graders. In response to a variety of questions concerning the definition of health, Natapoff found that children believe that health means feeling good, being able to engage in activities, and having no illness. Developmental findings were interpreted by this researcher to suggest that younger children, in comparison to older children, are less able to think analytically and abstractly about concepts such as health.

Campbell (1975), in a study of 264 children hospitalized with short-term illness, interviewed 6- to 12-year-olds concerning their concepts of illness. Results indicated significant developmental trends in illness concepts, including increasing complexity of concepts and increasing thematic content of the concepts. A group of 60 hospitalized 4- to 9-year-old children studied by Simeonsson et al. (1979) demonstrated similar Piagetian patterns.

In another related domain, Crider (1981) investigated children's understanding of their body physiology from a Piagetian perspective. She found that preschool children conceptualize their bodies in terms of global and observable activities. They are able to recognize some body parts (stomach, arms, bones, muscles) by their location on the body, but they do not understand their structure or function. By the preoperational stage, children are able to name a few organs and discuss their function in a rudimentary fashion. Children in the concrete operations stage possess specific knowledge of organs with respect to their shape, motion, and attributes. Later in this stage, children are able to understand transformations in the body (e.g., after lungs breathe in clean air, they breathe out dirty air). Finally, in preadolescence and adolescence (formal operations), the ability to organize body processes and functions in terms of differentiated transformations is achieved.

In a more recent examination of children's understanding of the biology of human bodies, children were queried about biological processes associated with breathing and eating (Toyamo, 2000). Children aged 4–8 years of age were able to state, when asked, that biological damage results from lack of breathing and eating. In a subsequent experiment by the same researcher, children were presented with multiple alternate explanations of what food and air are like inside bodies. All children reported that air would acquire warmth and color while inside bodies, but only the older children (aged 7 and 8 years) understood the biological transformation of food inside bodies. The younger children (aged 4 and 5 years) accepted the idea that food undergoes a transformation necessary for growth and health, but only some of them recognized the contribution of the sun to digestive processes for plants but not for mammals. These findings beg the question of the extent to which and at what developmental stages children can have theorylike understandings of biological processes such as digestion.

Piagetian stage theory has been used by Margaret and David Steward (1981) to analyze yet another aspect of children's health understanding: children's concepts of medical procedures. Three dimensions are identified: the "body–instrument interaction" (in which a child perceives the body as being impacted by an instrument such as a scale or a dialysis machine), the social role relationships between the child and the medical personnel, and the purpose of the procedure in terms of how it affects health. According to these researchers, preschool children engage in magical thinking about medical procedures. Medical personnel are imbued with absolute authority and are identified by perceptual cues (e.g., white coat, stethoscope). The purposes of procedures to children of this age are independent of health status. As they get older, children develop static and nonreversible cognitions about procedures. By the concrete operational stage, children are able to identify procedures and classify them as evaluative or therapeutic, although they may interpret them very literally and cannot understand deviance in the sequences involved in medical procedures. They are still respectful of medical authority but are more cognizant of the chain of command within medical personnel (e.g., the doctors are "in charge" of the nurses). With formal operational thought, it is possible for children to organize multiple procedures and their functions, defining the relative efficacy of each. At this point, it is understood that the authority of medical personnel depends on the compliance of the patient.

One additional area concerning children's age-related understanding of health-related concepts is children's beliefs about the long-term effects of alcohol and cocaine. In a study of over 200 children aged 6–12 years of age, Sigelman and her colleagues (Sigelman, Leach, Mack, & Bridges, 2000) found that age-related differentiation of the effects of alcohol, cocaine, and tobacco was limited but did increase with age.

The Piagetian stage model approach to understanding children's concepts of health and illness has been challenged. Specifically, most of the work derived from the Piagetian model of children's health knowledge and understanding has been generated from clinical interviews, mostly with sick and/or hospitalized children, with little attention paid to reliability, validity, and the development of instruments that could be used comparatively across studies. Moreover, the criteria used to determine children's cognitive stage often vary from study to study. These studies usually do not include control groups, confuse developmental status with age, and most often tap children's knowledge about serious illness rather than wellness (Burbach & Peterson, 1986; Eiser, 1989).

Eiser (1989) suggests that non-Piagetian models of cognitive development may be more appropriate for understanding children's cognitions about health and illness. Specifically, she offers script theory (Nelson, 1986) and Carey's (1985) model of conceptual change as alternative theoretical models to explain children's attitudes about health and illness. Nelson's (1986) script theory argues that children develop scriptlike, sequential representations of everyday, commonplace events such as going to the store or eating breakfast. Children may organize health events such as going to the doctor in such a manner, and may be able to recall and order specific consequences that occur within these events (Eiser, 1989; Garvey & Berndt, 1977). Two recent studies substantiate these ideas. Although these studies were undertaken for another purpose, namely, to provide data concerning children's suggestibility when functioning as witnesses, they suggest that script theory may be useful in elucidating children's health knowledge. Baker-Ward, Gordon, Ornstein, Larus, and Clubb (1993) studied young children's accuracy in recalling a pediatric examination over delays of as long as 6 weeks. Children aged 3, 5, and 7 years were questioned concerning their recall of the examination procedures. Results indicated that the younger children (aged 3 and 5) forgot more details that the 7-year-old children, but overall, all children demonstrated an impressive ability to remember a fairly detailed description of the exam procedures even 6 weeks after the exam. A second study, by Bruck and her associates (Bruck, Ceci, Francoeur, & Barr, 1995), examined 6-year-old children's ability to remember the amount of pain they suffered from and how much they cried after receiving a diphtheria, pertussis, tetanus (DPT) inoculation at their pediatrician's office 1 week after receiving one of three types of suggestive feedback: that the shot hurt, that the shot did not hurt, or that the shot was over. Results indicated that the suggestive feedback did not affect the children's recollections of pain or crying after the 1-week delay. In a follow-up, the investigators recontacted the children approximately 1 year later. At this point, some children were given suggestive feedback three times over a 2-week period; they were told they acted brave during the inoculation and did not cry. The other children received no feedback. Furthermore, in an elegant between-subjects crossed design, some children were given false information about the inoculator and others were given false information about the pediatrician. Results of this follow-up demonstrated some effects of the false information. The authors posited that three factors combined to weaken the children's memories after 1 year: the length of time between the inoculation and the follow-up suggestions, interference with the original suggestive feedback due to distress associated with the inoculation, and the repetition of the follow-up suggestive feedback over three sessions. Although these final results do suggest that children's recall of medical events may not be perfect, the Bruck et al. (1995) study and partial results from the second study indicate impressive recall of young children with respect to health events. Strong, consistent, and delayed suggestive feedback was necessary to disrupt these children's memories. This research underscores the potential of script theory to further illuminate children's developmental understanding of health.

Carey (1985) considers children's intuitive theories of behavior. Although this model of development suggests that children's knowledge increases as they age, Carey argues that children's understanding is unconstrained by structure. With respect to children's understanding of health, Carey's theory could be applied by tracing children's concepts of health from preschoolers' explanations of human body functioning in terms of wants and beliefs to preadolescents' "intuitive" biological understanding of the importance of human body functioning for the maintenance of life (Au, Romo, & DeWitt, 1999; Eiser, 1989; Hergenrather & Rabinowitz, 1991).

A Vygotskian perspective may also illuminate the relations between children's cognitive development and health socialization (Lees & Tinsley, 1998; Vygotsky, Rieber, & Carton, 1987). For young children, parents create supported learning situations in which their children can extend their skills and knowledge to a higher level of competence (Rogoff, 1997). The parents' involvement in this process, known as *scaffolding*, is described in six stages: (1) gaining the child's interest, (2) simplifying the tasks by reducing the number of steps for problem solution to a reasonable, manageable number, (3) motivating the child to maintain interest and participation in the task, (4) noting important discrepancies between the child's task performance and the ideal solution, (5) controlling frustration and risk, and (6) modeling the idealized version of the act. Each of these steps implies that the parent is acting in response to the child's progress and revising the scaffolding to respond to the child's accomplishments. This process can be applied to the way in which children learn any number of novel tasks, including but not limited to health and safety behaviors such as toothbrushing, food selection, and caring for minor injuries.

Although little data exist to validate the usefulness of these alternate theories for understanding children's concepts of health, these models suggest intriguing alternatives for conceptualizing developmental patterns in health understanding. However, given the limited predictive relation between knowledge and behavior, the extent to which models of children's health understanding are useful for illuminating the development of children's health-related behavior is questionable. While it seems apparent that children's understanding of illness and other health concepts does evolve in a systematic and predictable sequence, perhaps consistent with Piaget's theory of cognitive development (see Burbach & Peterson, 1986, and Gochman, 1988, 1997, for detailed reviews of this literature), individual differences also exist in children's understanding of health.

Individual Differences in Children's Health Attitudes

A second focus of the research on children's health attitudes and behavior is on individual differences in these areas, as reflected in such constructs as health locus of control that, in turn, have been demonstrated to relate to children's health behavior and health outcomes. An individual differences perspective on children's acquisition of health-related attitudes and behavior, in contrast to a Piagetian stage model, shifts the focus from discovering a maturational unfolding of abilities in these domains to the personality, social, and cultural variables that mediate this acquisition.

Research in the individual differences tradition in children's health attitudes and behavior has focused on two areas: children's perceived vulnerability to health problems and children's health motivation. Several researchers have conceptualized children's health motivation as children's beliefs concerning their control of their health (Parcel & Meyer, 1978). The Children's Health Locus of Control Scale, modeled after the adult Multidimensional Health Locus of Control Scales (Wallston, Wallston, Smith, & Dobbins, 1987), is composed of three factors: (1) internal control, (2) powerful others, and (3) chance control. This scale has been used to assess the results of a preschool health intervention program (Parcel, Bruhn, & Murray, 1984).

Based on prior research concerning the general predictive relation between health knowledge and health attitudes, it would be hypothesized that children whose health attitudes are characterized by greater control of their health (i.e., internal health locus of control) would access more information about health and be more knowledgeable concerning health. There is evidence that this is the case. The more internally a child scored on a locus of control measure, the more sophisticated were the clues he or she used to identify sickness or health (Neuhauser, Amsterdam, Hines, & Steward, 1978). Similarly, children (5–16 years old) with internally related health beliefs had more sophisticated conceptual understandings of disease than children with externally oriented health beliefs. Healthy children were more sophisticated in their knowledge about illness and were more internal in their health locus of control than children with chronic illnesses, suggesting that children's health locus of control may, to some extent, mediate their developing concepts of wellness and illness (Sanger, Sandler, & Perrin, 1988). However, it is clear that more work in this area is necessary. In children with insulin-dependent diabetes, higher levels of disease knowledge corresponded to more external locus of control beliefs, although this finding held for boys only (Hamburg & Inoff, 1982).

Another area of research on children's health attitudes has focused on children's perceived vulnerability to health problems. Gochman (1987) performed a series of studies utilizing the Gochman Perceived Vulnerability Scale, which assesses the extent to which children perceive the likelihood of experiencing selected health problems. Results of these studies indicated that perceived vulnerability increases between the ages of 8 and 13 and decreases thereafter, although these shifts are relative in the sense that children's overall perceived health vulnerability is low

(Gochman, 1987). Other results suggest that childhood perceived health vulnerability is consistent within children over time and is related to self-concept and self-esteem. However, there has been no attempt to relate these issues to childhood health behavior and health. Gochman (1987) has also studied children's health motivation. The data from these studies indicate that health is not a very significant value or priority for children, especially for those younger than 9 years of age. However, there has been no attempt to relate these issues to childhood health behavior and health status.

Integrating Stage Theory and Individual Differences
Perspectives on Children's Health Attitudes and Behavior

These two viewpoints on children's health attitudes and behavior, the Piagetian stage theory and the individual differences perspective, are not necessarily incompatible. Piagetian stage theory, as applied to children's understanding of health-related concepts, focuses on the structure and content of children's thought on these issues in much the same way that developmental psychologists studying children's understanding of health follow a determined, relatively invariant developmental course and minimize within-stage variability in children's conceptualizations of health. Researchers who study children's health attitudes and behavior within the latter framework attempt to describe the normative progression of children's health knowledge.

An individual differences viewpoint, based on a psychometric tradition in psychology, focuses on variability in children's health attitudes and behavior. Personality dimensions, as well as social and nonsocial environmental factors that explain children's health attitudes and behavior, are studied with an emphasis on children's within-age/stage variability.

The integration of these two perspectives in the study of children's health knowledge, attitudes, and behavior is an important goal in this area. Within the cognitive tradition, even though it is assumed that socialization is a factor in the development of children's knowledge, the role of these variables has been minimized in traditional stage theory explications of children's health attitudes and behavior. Similarly, most researchers who examine children's health attitudes and behavior from an individual differences perspective do not adequately acknowledge the cognitive developmental constraints in children's understanding that are relevant to the personality variables considered (Nicholls & Miller, 1983). Researchers who have simultaneously utilized both stage and individual differences perspectives offer unique glimpses of children's health understanding. For example, Neuhauser and colleagues (Neuhauser et al., 1978) found that children 8 years of age and older with a stronger internal locus of control are better able to recognize illness symptoms than other children.

Children's Health Attitudes and Their Relation to Children's Health Behavior

The role of health attitudes in children's preventive health behavior is an important factor. Recent evidence suggests that although U.S. children do know about some aspects of healthy diet, home safety, and the dangers associated with tobacco, alcohol, and other drug use, that knowledge is not reflected in their behavior. In a survey of over 3,000 children between the ages of 6 and 12 years, children's awareness of healthy behavior was not matched by their self-reported actual health behavior. For example, while almost 86% of the children stated that they should eat fruits and vegetables at least three times per day, almost 50% responded that they ate only one fruit or one vegetable or neither the day before (American Health Foundation, 1995).

One study demonstrated moderate relations between health knowledge, health beliefs, and avoidance of risk behaviors in a sample of 6- to 17-year-olds (Radius, Dillman, Becker, Rosenstock, & Horvath, 1980). Interestingly, only about one-half of the adolescents in this sample reported worrying about health at all, and only about one-third reported personal accountability for health. Two studies of adolescents' beliefs about illness susceptibility, illness severity, and effectiveness of action and their relations to health behaviors demonstrated few relations between these domains (Kegeles & Lund, 1982; Weisenberg, Kegeles, & Lund, 1980). In these studies, the health attitudes of junior high school students were measured before and after the introduction of a dental program. Practically no relations were found between these students' attitudes (either before or after the program) and health behavior. However, it is unclear whether there are actually few relations between children's health attitudes and behavior in these studies or whether possibly, as the authors suggest, the nonfindings may have been due to the specific outcome behavior (i.e., obtaining topical fluoride applications in school) being subject to influence from teachers and/or peers rather than to children's own personal health attitudes. It is conceivable that there was a mismatch between the specificity of the attitudes targeted for change and the outcome variable measured to document the change. The ambiguity of these findings, in light of other work reporting child health attitude–behavior links, further suggests the importance of additional work investigating the relations between children's health-related attitudes and behavior using a wider range of health behaviors.

There is some evidence to substantiate the role of children's health attitudes in determining children's illness behaviors (illness behaviors are a subcategory of children's health behaviors). In a study of fourth- and eighth-grade students, Mechanic (1965) found that a majority of boys and girls in both age categories reported that they had no fear of getting hurt and that they did not pay attention to pain. Pain denial and risk-taking were higher among eighth- than fourth-grade children, both boys and girls. Professing willingness to report symptoms of illness was not related to age or sex except among the eighth-grade boys, nearly half of whom reported that they would not report illness. Mechanic interpreted these data to suggest that boys learn to deny pain and illness, although an alternate explanation is that boys may report pain only to selected persons. However, this study does not provide data on the children's actual illness behavior, but only on what the children reported that they did.

In summary, additional work on the relations between children's health-related attitudes and behavior is necessary to further clarify this area. As is characteristic of the general psychological literature establishing links between attitudes and behavior, the evidence is mixed (Pratkanis, Breckler, & Greenwald, 1989). Additional research is needed to specify these relations, with greater attention paid to structuring the specificity of both the health attitudes and behavior under consideration to be parallel, and acknowledgment that parents remain the mediators of much of children's health behavior.

Children's Health Behavior

Descriptions of young children's personal behaviors associated with seeking medical attention and health maintenance are rare. Young children's routine or preventive health care visits are manifestations of parents' health behaviors. For the most part, except for child-initiated school health office visits, preschool-age and school-age children are taken to practitioners by adults when the children are perceived by adults to have an illness or injury requiring professional attention. Children's self-initiated care occurs only under unusual circumstances. This is consonant with more general theories concerning parents' management of children's lives and the distinction between parent-initiated child behavior and child-initiated behavior (Hartup & Stevens, 1999).

A Special Case of Children's Health Behavior: Children's School Nurse Visits

One group of studies has examined a specific facet of children's health behavior: children's self-initiated visits to school health offices. The frequency of visits by high school students to the school health office was studied by Rogers and Reese (1965). Over a 9-month period, over half of the boys and more than two-thirds of the girls visited the health office at least once, and 1 student in 20 visited more than 7 times. A high frequency of health office visits was related to high absence rates, smoking, and low achievement. Rates of health office utilization remained constant in these children in subsequent years.

Lewis and Lewis (1982) conducted a longitudinal study of visits to the school health office among elementary school students. In their study, children visited the health office without adult permission. Results indicated that a very small percentage of the children (15%) accounted for 50% of all of the visits and that approximately one-quarter of the children never visited the health office.

Other studies of school health office visits are also of interest. Stamler and Palmer (1971) studied the relation between elementary school-age children's visits to the health office and ratings of dependence of the children. Although the study had sampling problems, the results indicated that children who frequently visited the health office also had high dependency ratings. Van Arsdell, Roghmann, and Nader (1972) demonstrated that among Euro-American students, girls visited the health office more than boys, and that dependency and rates of visitation were positively correlated and peer acceptance, grades, achievement scores, and high rates of visitation were negatively correlated.

In summary, the literature documenting patterns in children's visits to school health offices suggests that some children visit at a fairly high rate and that a minority of students visit at a very high rate. Moreover, it is apparent that children who frequently visit the school health office are characterized by high dependence, low academic achievement, and low peer status relative to children who utilize these services less frequently.

To summarize, children's health attitudes and behavior have been studied with a cognitive-structural approach and, to a lesser extent, by examining individual difference factors in this domain. Both approaches contribute to our understanding of how children learn and are socialized about health. The relations among children's attitudes about health and children's health behavior have also been examined.

Several issues remain to be addressed if further significant progress is to occur in this research area. One issue is further delineation of the mechanisms involved in translating children's health attitudes into health behavior. Next steps in elucidating childhood socialization of health attitudes and behavior involve an exploration of the ways in which children's health attitudes translated into health behavior can be explained by existing theories of concept formation (e.g., Carey, 1985; Eiser, 1989; Markman, 1989). In this case, children's understanding of health progresses via a naive biological understanding that becomes more complex as children age and could be the basis for children's health behavior.

A second hypothesis is that children's health behavioral patterns are governed by scripts (Eiser, 1989; Nelson, 1986). This hypothesis suggests that children learn rituals of health behavior (e.g., toothbrushing, exercise, wearing a seat belt in a moving car). These rituals or scripts, and the behaviors included in them, become more detailed and specific as children age, and the behaviors become context bound.

Other approaches may also be of value in accounting for children's health behavior, such as a social information processing model (Bandura, 1989; Crick & Dodge, 1994). Social information processing theorists believe that behavior is dependent on the interpretation of social cues present in a situation. As applied to health, this theory assumes that children enter each situation with a data base of past health-related experiences and a health goal of some sort (e.g., avoiding tooth decay, normalizing body weight). When an event occurs that requires explanation (e.g., illness), these theorists propose that children's response to the situation and the social cues it provides depend on a series of cognitive steps. These steps involve gathering information about the event, interpreting the event, considering alternative behaviors (e.g., tell the mother, go to bed), and deciding to actually report the symptoms of illness to the mother. Research has demonstrated that children exhibit individual differences in both past experiences and information processing skills. Thus, children with varying illness histories might be expected to react differently to symptoms of illness, and children with differing levels of information processing skills may vary in the ability to perceive and interpret health symptoms or to identify, choose, and enact alternative health behaviors. Although this model explains variations in children's health-related information processing skills, it does not address the issue of how children come to be more or less skillful at processing health-related information or why children have different information processing styles. Moreover, the extent to which child personality characteristics or familial socialization impacts these skills is unclear. However, a social-cognitive approach may be useful in generating new insights with respect to translating children's health attitudes into health behavior.

3

Parents' Health Beliefs

Parents influence their children's health through a variety of mechanisms, including their beliefs and behavior. This chapter will examine how parents' beliefs and behavior affect children's health attitudes, behavior, and outcomes.

Parents' Health Beliefs

Studies of parents' attitudes and beliefs suggest that parental socialization practices are guided by parents' attitudes toward and understanding of child development and behavior (cf. Grusec, Goodnow, & Kuczynski, 2000; Sigel & Dorval, 2000) within cultural contexts (Harkness & Keefer, 2000). Data supporting these relations are found most prominently in the domains of cognitive development (Miller, 2000; Sigel & Dorval, 2000) and social development (Simpkins & Parke, 2001). However, a major way in which parents influence children's health is related to their attitudes about health, and usually function via their influence on parents' behavior rather than by interaction with the child (Loveland-Cherry, Leech, Laetz, & Dielman, 1996). Studies of parents' attitudes and beliefs concerning their children's health suggest that these are important factors in parents' health behavior on behalf of their children and their socialization of children's health behavior. Parental behaviors on behalf of children's health and supervision of their children's health-related behaviors seem to reflect the parental caregiving role and parental control of many aspects of young children's behavior (Hartup, 1979). Lau and his colleagues (Lau, Quadrel, & Hartman, 1990) found that mothers influenced their children either indirectly, through the transmission of health beliefs, or directly through explicit training in four areas of health behavior: exercise, diet, alcohol use, and seat belt use.

Parents' beliefs and behavior may be transmitted unintentionally to their children, or they may be transferred in the context of training children to engage in health behavior (Lau et al., 1990). Consider the ideas of Ellen, mother of 4-year-old Rachel, when she was asked why Rachel is sometimes ill. "Mothers don't want for their children to get sick, and do everything possible to prevent it, but sometimes children just get sick. In some cases, you just cannot do anything about it." In this statement, Rachel's mother demonstrates several aspects of parents' attitudes about health that have been demonstrated to affect children's health behavior and actual health. She tells us that she values Rachel's wellness, but more importantly, she communicates her maternal health locus of control or her beliefs concerning the controllability of Rachel's health and mothers' role in controllability. Next, we examine current research that focuses on these issues.

Parents' Value of Health

Usually, the value that parents place on their children's health is examined in the context of the value that parents place on other goals for their children. These include education, prosperity, peace, and friendship/companionship. Parents are asked to rank several goals with respect to the importance they place on their children's attaining these goals. In general, researchers using this strategy find, not surprisingly, that parents rank their children's health very highly in this context.

Studies of the value that parents place on children's health demonstrate that these beliefs can also be expressed in parents' health behavior on behalf of their children. For example, in our laboratory, we found that women who valued their children's health the most were the ones most likely to obtain prenatal health services with the greatest reliability and conformance with their physicians' recommended schedule for prenatal health visits. Evaluations of the value that adults generally place on health (relative to other life values) have yielded equivocal results. When the health perceptions of adults were examined, participants in this study ranked health, on average, higher than the other 17 of Rokeach's (1974) life values (e.g., inner harmony, self-respect, sense of accomplishment, freedom), although approximately 30% of them did not rank health among their first 5 values. Lau, Hartman, and Ware (1986) developed and utilized a four-item Likert scale focused specifically on health value.

Results from the use of this scale with five populations differing in age and health status suggest that the value placed on health varies by gender, age, and educational status. Specifically, reports of the value placed on their children's health by parents are very rare. Although Lau et al. (1986) used the health value scale described previously to compare the health value of adolescent girls and their parents (results suggested that parents value health to a greater extent than do their daughters), this scale measured parents' value of health in general, which is not necessarily synonymous with the value they place on health with respect to their children.

Other Parental Health Beliefs

In an investigation of the relation between the health beliefs of mothers and their children, Dielman and colleagues found that mothers' and children's perceptions of the seriousness of and susceptibility to disease were significantly linked (Dielman et al., 1982; Rubovits & Wolynn, 1999). Other recent research illuminates the significant impact of parents' perceptions of their children's health vulnerability. Thomasgard and Metz (1995) reviewed research findings on the vulnerable child syndrome, which is characterized by increased parental perceptions of a child's vulnerability to illness or injury, which are either real or feared. Although the ways in which these parental perceptions of child vulnerability are translated into children's emotional, cognitive, and social deficits are unclear, they are related to children's school underachievement, child psychosomatic illness, and increased use of pediatric health care services. Other studies of parental anxiety about children's health status confirm the relation between parental anxiety and parents' health behavior on behalf of their children. Hatcher and colleagues (Hatcher, Powers, & Richtsmeier, 1993) found that parents who experienced more anxiety about their infants' illness symptoms were more likely to seek pediatric health care than were less anxious parents. Moreover, several studies have demonstrated that anxious parents do not demonstrate good judgment about the severity of their children's illness (Bauchner, McCarthy, Sznajderman, & Baron, 1987), tend to have a poor perception of their children's condition, and may misinterpret information provided during a pediatric visit (Richtsmeier & Hatcher, 1994). These studies highlight the importance of parents' perceptions and beliefs about their children's health status in the use of parents as informants about their children's health and in the deliverance of health information about children to parents by health professionals.

Another area in which parents' health attitudes appear to significantly affect children's health is parents' attitudes toward medication (Ranelli, Bartsch, & London, 2000). Maiman and her colleagues (Maiman, Becker, & Katlic, 1986) found that mothers' perceptions concerning their children's susceptibility to health problems and the effectiveness of non-prescription medications were related to possessing and using a greater number of categories of medication. In addition, possession and use of over-the-counter medications were positively associated with mothers' perception that their family had more illnesses and their perception of control. Similarly, Bush and Iannotti (1988) found moderate agreement between mothers and their elementary school children in their health beliefs concerning medicine use. Later interviews of a subset of these children and mothers revealed stability across a 3-year period.

Ideas about influencing children's safety from unintentional injuries is another area in which parental health beliefs affect children. Valsiner and Lightfoot (1987) suggest that parents or other caregivers engage in childhood risk management on behalf of their children to the extent that their beliefs about cultural norms, and characteristics of their children and other children, allow them to perceive an understanding of the risk of any given situation for their children. These authors believe that the "trans-action between the environment, the child, and the caregiver" (p. 71) determines the risk associated with children's behavior. Parents use their knowledge and beliefs about such factors as the appropriateness of dangers, possible preventive actions, children's goals, and the setting to engage in decision making about whether to preempt children's actions. The parents' ability to reason about these aspects of children's safety guides their parenting behavior.

Parents' beliefs about health affect their health behavior not only on behalf of abled children but on behalf of disabled children as well. Affleck and his colleagues have studied how mothers' beliefs about children's disabilities affect maternal behavior. Results of these studies indicate that mothers who blame others for their child's developmental disability are more likely to have caregiving problems and to be less sensitive to their children than mothers who accept at least partial responsibility for their child's condition (Affleck, McGrade, Allen, & McQueeney, 1985).

Another area in which parents' beliefs about children's health appear to be very powerful in determining their health behavior on behalf of their children is injury prevention. Peterson and her colleagues (Peterson, Farmer, & Kashani, 1990) utilized a health belief model to predict parental teaching of safety skills and unintentional injury prevention. Results indicated that the more parents felt they knew about safety, the more confident they felt about intervening to prevent children's injuries. In turn, parents who perceived interventions to be effective in preventing childhood injuries reported more attempts at teaching their children to avoid behavior that would render them susceptible to injury. Although these findings are not related to actual childhood injury levels, they suggest further avenues for investigating the relations between parents' health beliefs, parents' health behavior on behalf of children, and children's health behavior.

One interesting way in which parents' beliefs about health have been explored is through a developmental analysis of how seriously parents view children's symptom reporting and complaining. Wilkinson (1988) has intensively studied parents' reactions to their children's illness complaints, with particular interest in how and when parents decide that a child is pretending to be ill. He relates the criteria by which parents decide how seriously to take the complaints: (1) alterations in children's behavior patterns, particularly their daily routines such as waking up and eating; (2) reluctance to attend day care or school; and (3) mood or appearance. None of the parents in Wilkinson's sample labeled a child's behavior as pretending to be ill before the age of 8 years. Wilkinson's interviews with 8- to 13-year-old children demonstrated that they had an understanding of how their parents interpret their symptom reporting, which permitted them to engage in deceit about illness. Wilkinson reports, "Generally these ... children could adopt roles both at home and at school which made the discrimination between play and non-play situations [about illness] much more difficult for those around them" (1988, p. 180). In interviews with the parents of these children, Wilkinson found interesting socialization strategies that the parents employed to teach their children the "rules" of illness reporting. For example, he reports the moral rules about claiming a stomachache that one family established:

> We never play with situations which are serious.
> Tummy ache is always a serious illness complaint.
> Therefore any messages about tummy ache must be interpreted within non-play frames. (p. 182)

Wilkinson found that by the time their children were 8 years old, parents believed that their children had the ability to pretend to be ill, and that they used illness complaints to "negotiate their status" (p. 183), that is, stay home from school, be allowed to watch daytime television, be relieved of household chores, and so on. These investigations are useful and remind us that parents' interpretation of children's health behavior may have as much salience or even more salience for parental behavior on behalf of their children's health than the children's behaviors themselves.

Health Locus of Control Beliefs

Adult health locus of control and explanatory style have been used to explain and predict various adult health attitude and behavior domains (Peterson & Seligman, 1987; Wallston, Wallston, Smith, & Dobbins, 1987). There have been a number of investigations of the relation between parents' health attitudes with respect to their own health in general and their children's health status. Outcome measures employed in these studies are usually parent-provided health-related products or services obtained for children, including well-child variables such as vitamin usage (Gossler, 1980), child restraint/seat belt usage (Guske, 1980), and immunization levels (Berger, 1980) and ill-child variables such as recovery from an illness, compliance with medical regimens, and utilization of medical care (Becker & Green, 1975; Campbell, 1978; DeVellis, DeVellis, Revicki, Lurie, Runyan, & Bristol, 1986; Drotar, 1981; Levenson, Copeland, Morrow, Pfefferbaum, & Silberberg, 1983; Mechanic, 1980). However, the results of these studies have been disappointing. Two studies found relations between mothers' own health attitudes and children's health outcomes. Becker, Maiman, Kirscht, Haefner and Drachman (1977) found that mothers' general and specific attitudes with respect to their own health in terms of vulnerability, severity, benefits of change, and barriers to health were related to subsequent weight loss by their children. However, these relations may be significant because the actions of the parent (i.e., determination of the child's diet) guide the child's behavior (i.e., content of food eaten). With the exception of this study by Becker and his colleagues, the findings that generally indicate that mothers' health attitudes are unrelated to children's health may be due to the fact that the health locus of control scales used in all these studies measured the *mothers' perceptions of control over their own health, not control over the health of their children.* In summary, although it would be theoretically expected that mothers' attitudes concerning their own health locus of control should be related to health behavior on behalf of their children, the findings generally suggest that this may be the case in only limited ways. Several groups of researchers have attempted more successfully to relate parents' health locus of control to their health behavior on behalf of their children by choosing a slightly different focus: parents' attitudes concerning their control over their children's health in contrast to their perceptions of control over their own health.

Maiman and her colleagues (Maiman, Becker, & Katlic, 1985, 1986) examined the relation between mothers' attitudes concerning medication use and mothers' use of medications for treating children's symptoms. A sample of 500 mothers of children 2–12 years of age were surveyed, during well-child care, concerning their possession and use of nonprescription medications for their children. Results suggest that mothers' attitudes are important in understanding their medication behavior on behalf of their children. Mothers' perceptions concerning their children's susceptibility to health problems and the effectiveness of nonprescription medications were related to possessing and using more types of medications. In addition, possession and use of over-the-counter medications was positively associated with mothers' perception that their family had more illnesses and with their perception of control. Although this study clearly demonstrates the determinants of mothers' home medication supply and use with children, it does not explain how these attitudes are translated into parents' health behavior on behalf of their children. DeVellis et al. (1986) have developed and validated the Child Improvement Locus of Control (CILC) scales. Two groups of parents, with autistic children and with physically ill children, completed questionnaires measuring their attitudes toward chance, divine influence, professional help, their child, and themselves as factors influencing their child's improvement. Results indicated that parents' attitudes toward influences on their child increased with the child's age and the belief in external factors (chance and divine influence) and was greater among African American parents; in addition, their belief in parental influence decreased with illness severity. However, these studies do not relate these parental attitudes to parental health-related behavior on behalf of children.

Tinsley has completed a series of studies investigating the relations among mothers' attitudes concerning the control they perceive with respect to their children's health, utilization of prenatal or childhood preventive health services, and children's health (Tinsley & Holtgrave, 1989; Howell-Koren, & Tinsley 1990; Tinsley, Trupin, Owens, & Boyum, 1993). The results of these studies suggest that mothers' perception of their control over their children's perinatal and pediatric outcomes is related to their use of prenatal and pediatric services, which in turn is related to children's health outcomes. Specifically, mothers' belief in their control of their infants' health was positively related to utilization of prenatal and pediatric care, and children who received this care had a better perinatal and pediatric health status. Studies of other types of maternal health beliefs, focused on the value mothers place on their children's health and the subsequent effect these attitudes have on maternal behavior, also demonstrate that maternal health beliefs can be expressed in maternal health behavior on behalf of children.

Parents from different cultures may have varying beliefs about the causes of wellness and illness and transmit these beliefs to their children (Harkness & Keefer, 2000). Euro-American mothers often perceive a direct scientific cause-and-effect relationship between biological problems and child development. Mothers from other ethnic groups often place a strong emphasis on fate, bad luck, sins of parents, foods the mother eats, or evil spirits as the causative factors in children's health status (Hanson, Lynch, & Wayman, 1990). These perceptions affect the way in which children's health is viewed within families and cultures and the types of health services mothers are willing to utilize on behalf of their children's health. For example, in an interview study of Mexican mothers of infants with handicaps, Gault (1990) found that 93% of the mothers attributed the child's handicap to the mothers' experiencing a "big fright" during pregnancy. Additional studies underscore the importance of understanding parents' culturally influenced beliefs about health. In an investigation of the causes and symptoms of children's illness among Guatemalan mothers, researchers found that Western biomedical models of illness causation are relatively irrelevant, or at best coexist with more culture-specific traditional explanations of childhood respiratory illnesses and diarrhea (Pebley, Hurtado, & Goldman, 1999).

Other research confirms that health-related stereotypes are culturally related and transmitted from mother to child. Olvera-Ezzell and her colleagues (Olvera-Ezzell, Power, & Cousins, 1990) found significant concordance in the judgments of weight-related physical attractiveness in obese and normal-weight Mexican American mothers and their 7- to 12-year-old daughters. Several studies suggest similar parent–child socialization of preference for body builds (Adams, Hicken, & Salehi, 1988). Thus, although there is solid evidence that mothers' health beliefs influence their health behavior on behalf of their children, the mechanisms by which this occurs have not been well explored.

Fiese and Sameroff (1989) have identified a number of family beliefs that affect child health, which they term the *family code*. They define the family code as a system of family definitions that are used as guidelines for the family's behavior, including family paradigms (core assumptions, convictions, or beliefs that each family member holds), family stories and myths, and family rituals (Reiss, 1989). As discussed previously, mothers' beliefs about children's health have a substantial impact on their health behavior on behalf of their on children and, in turn, on children's health outcomes. Family stories and myths illuminate how individual family members, or the family as a whole, interpret and manage health-related experiences and events (Reisch, Tinsley & Phillips, 1994). For example, a mother who believes that her children have fewer colds than other children because "angels are protecting them" presents a different pediatric anticipatory guidance opportunity than a mother who recounts her numerous and continuing efforts to protect her children from infectious diseases through good nutrition and hygiene. Finally, family rituals appear to provide, at least in some cases, some buffering from the negative aspects of a family member's poor health. Wertlieb, Hauser, and Jacobson (1986) found that maintaining regular routines and engaging in social and recreational activities as a family helped to avoid behavioral problems in families with a child with diabetes. These findings provide strong support for the ways in which maternal beliefs, in the context of the family, affect child health symptom perception and health services usage.

Parents' Beliefs and Children's Outcomes

Parents' beliefs may directly impact children's behaviors and outcomes (Miller, 2000). Parents' beliefs may directly affect children, for example, by influencing the manner in which parents construct the child's environment, or by affecting general expectations of parents that are conveyed to children through their cumulative history of interaction, rather than by particular parenting acts or behaviors (Miller, 2000). For example, a child may come to realize that her parents value independence in simple health care behaviors such as toothbrushing and seat belt use, even though her parents have not communicated that message through any specific behavior or statement.

In fact, a path analysis (McGillicuddy-DeLisi, 1992) found empirical support for a direct path of influence from parents' beliefs about children's constructivist nature to children's competence that was not moderated by maternal behaviors. This finding supports the hypothesis that parent belief systems about child development exert a strong influence on child outcomes that is only partially visible as parenting behaviors. Thus, in order to understand the manner in which parents socialize children's health behaviors, one must look beyond overt parenting behaviors and styles to examine other influences of parental belief systems. Bacon and Ashmore (1985) described a detailed model of the multiple ways in which parents' cognitions and beliefs influence their interactions with their children. Following is a description of their model and its relevance for parental health socialization.

Cognitive-Affective Structure of Parental Cognition

Just as they do with their other experiences, parents organize and categorize the behavior of their children so as to simplify response categories. Thus, the cognitive activities of parents are essential variables that intervene between the behavior stream of their child and their own socializing response. Bacon and Ashmore (1985) posited a cognitive-affective framework to explain the role of parental cognitions in socialization. According to these authors, four parental cognitive-affective structures influence parents' responses to their child: (1) long- and short-term goals, (2) affect and belief systems, (3) spatial models, and (4) perceptual and motor skills. Long-term goals are some of the most important cognitive and affective structures of parents. There are two long-term goals: (1) to protect the child from harm and (2) to socialize the child. Of these long-term goals, the first is more powerful (Bacon & Ashmore, 1985). The impetus to protect one's child from harm can be seen as a critical aspect of parental behavior in the health domain. This goal operates in parents' search for both acute and preventive health care for their children (Lees & Tinsley, 1998). The second long-term goal, socialization, is defined as the parents' motive to guide children's behavior so that they become accepted members of society. Specifically, the socialization of health behavior involves teaching and guiding the child's health behaviors so that they conform to social and cultural norms. Bacon and Ashmore emphasized that these societal norms influence both the ways in which parents attend to their child's health behaviors and parents' responses to their child's health behaviors and activities.

The second cognitive and affective structure contains the affect and belief systems of parents. These systems are structured sets of knowledge about their child or childrearing, including general structured knowledge of the parent that impacts childrearing (e.g., political, economic, or religious beliefs), parents' implicit theories about childrearing, and parents' beliefs and feelings about each child's potential behavior patterns. Each of these affect and belief systems influences the manner in which parents respond to particular health or safety behaviors of their child (Lees & Tinsley, 1998).

The third group of cognitive and affective structures contains cognitive maps that specify levels of difficulty for a child according to his current developmental level. These cognitive-affective structures influence the way parents interpret the effectiveness of their child's activities and thereby affect parents' reaction to the child's behavior.

These three cognitive structures affect the parent's socialization of health behaviors (Tinsley & Lees, 1998). For example, the parent's general knowledge structures reflect cultural norms for the processes of certain health practices and timetables for demonstrating and teaching health behaviors. The parent's implicit childrearing theories impact on the manner in which the parent structures health behavior tasks, the type of reinforcement the parent utilizes, and the decisions the parent makes concerning when to turn over control of a health task or activity to the child, that is, when the child is developmentally ready to perform certain activities or tasks. Specific theories about each child also affect when and how the parent structures health tasks and learning situations for the child. A parent's cognitive map for a child describes where that parent must intervene in keeping the child healthy and where the child can maneuver alone.

The final category of cognitive-affective structures proposed by Bacon and Ashmore concerns the perceptual and motor skills of the parent. The parent's perceptual ability to discriminate between the behaviors of a sick child and a well child affects the parent's behavior. In addition, the parent of a young child may need to develop new motor skills (Tinsley & Lees, 1998).

Parents' Categorization of Children's Behavior

Some of the other cognitive activities of parents that affect their interactions with their child include the way in which the parents break up the behavior stream of the child into units, how they label those units, how they respond to the units, and how they organize or categorize the units (Bacon & Ashmore, 1986). For example, when a preschooler reaches for candy rather than a piece of fruit for a snack, the parent may see this either as an isolated unit of behavior or as part of a continuing stream of defiant behaviors. The parent may label the action in several different ways, each of which will affect the parent's response. The action may be labeled "Mary doesn't have enough sense to choose health snacks," or "Mary doesn't understand yet that candy is unhealthy," or "Mary always chooses candy because her friends eat it," or "Mary is doing this because she is trying to upset me and she knows this makes me angry."

Each of these labels for Mary's action is likely to result in a different kind of response from her parent – a different type of parental intervention (Tinsley & Lees, 1998).

In addition, the way in which a parent categorizes a child's behavior will have a significant effect on socialization processes. For example, a parent may categorize the refusal to wear a seat belt as either part of "a stage" or "she just wants attention." These two categorizations will result in very different parental responses. Thus, the manner in which parents socialize their children's health beliefs and behaviors is clearly related to parents' beliefs about children's health, as well as their control over their children's health.

4

Parents' Promotion of Their Children's Health

Childrearing: A Pathway Between Parents' Beliefs and Behavior

One pathway through which parent and child similarity in health beliefs may occur is through parental childrearing behavior. The classic study relating parents' childrearing behavior to children's health behavior was performed by Pratt (1973). This interview investigation of 273 families (mother, father, and 9- to 13-year-old children) involved assessing the relations between childrearing styles and child health behaviors (e.g., toothbrushing, exercise, nutritional practices). Pratt identified a style of parenting she termed the *energized family*, which was related to the highest levels of child health practices. The parents in these energized families gave their children a high degree of autonomy and used reasoning rather than punishment as a discipline strategy. Although most of the correlations were low, Pratt reported that childrearing practices had a significant effect on children's health behavior even when the parents' own health behaviors are controlled. Childrearing attitudes that recognized the child as an individual and fostered the child's assumption of responsibility were associated with positive health behavior in children (toothbrushing, good sleep habits, exercise, good nutritional practices, and refraining from smoking). In contrast, children raised in families with an autocratic style of childrearing were not as likely to practice such behaviors. The study was weakened by reliance on the children's perceptions of their parents' childrearing practices even when evidence from the parents themselves was available. Moreover, the independent contribution of mothers' childrearing practices, separately from those of fathers, was not examined separately. Four more recent studies confirm these relations between general childrearing practices and child health behavior.

Lau and Klepper (1988), in a study of the illness orientations of 6- to 12-year-old children, examined parents' childrearing practices. Parental punishment and control (i.e., frequency of spanking, frequency of isolation, parents' strictness, and the importance of discipline to parents) were found to influence children's self-esteem, approaching statistical significance. In turn, children's self-esteem was a significant predictor of their illness orientation.

Further validation of this work is found cross-ethnically (Harkness & Keefer, 2000). A series of studies of the nutrition-related motivational strategies of Mexican American mothers of 4- to 8-year-old children indicate that serving and helping children with their food was associated with food consumption compliance, and threats and bribes were negatively associated with healthy food consumption (see Birch, Marlin, & Rotter, 1984; Olvera-Ezzell et al., 1990). Yamasaki (1990), in a study of parental childrearing attitudes associated with Type A behaviors (characterized by high scores on time urgency, competitive achievement-striving, and aggressiveness-hostility, and identified as one of the factors leading to coronary heart disease) in Japanese preschool children, found that mothers of Type A boys were less anxious about them, less affectionate toward them, demanded more compliance of them, and were less concerned about them than mothers of Type B boys. Furthermore, mothers of Type A girls were less anxious about their daughters than were mothers of Type B girls.

Finally, a study by Lees and Tinsley (1998) provides additional evidence for the link between parental childrearing practices and children's health behavior. In this study, mothers' parenting behavior and children's health behavior were assessed in a sample of 70 preschool children. Results indicated that warm, nurturant mothers (those who gave higher than average amounts of verbal praise, hugs, and kisses as rewards for good behavior) had children who were more independent in a variety of health behaviors, such as toothbrushing, handwashing, exercising, going to bed at a regular time, and avoiding risk by staying away from poisons, as reported by parents. Additional results suggested that children whose mothers reported using monetary rewards and granting special privileges for good behavior had a tendency to make fewer nutritious food choices, as reported by their preschool teachers, than mothers who chose to use warmth and nurturance as strategies for encouraging good behavior in their children. In addition, mothers' general beliefs about childrearing were related to some of their children's safety behaviors. For example, mothers who reported that children should get more discipline than they usually receive reported that their children showed less independence in seat belt use, whereas mothers who believed that parents should be more flexible reported that their children exercised more independently. These findings seem to indicate some relation between maternal orientations toward child-oriented mothering styles and autonomous healthy behavior by their children, with a corresponding possible relation between authoritarian mothering and less independence in risk-preventive behaviors by their children.

In support of Pratt's findings about the value of rewarding children for their good behavior, our study found that the total time mothers reported using rewards for good behavior related to independence in taking naps and keeping regular bedtimes. Use of rewards was also related to less risky behavior, as reported by preschool teachers. These studies, considered together, suggest that non-health-specific childrearing behavior affects children's health behavior and illustrates the potential of this path from parental attitudes to parental behavior to child health behavior.

Together, these studies provide support for the hypothesis of parent–child transmission of health attitudes. Additional longitudinal work is necessary to clarify these relations. We now turn from an examination of the way in which parents' beliefs affect children's health orientation to another way in which parents influence their children's health attitudes and behavior: parents' health behavior.

Parents' Health Behavior

Social learning theory focuses on the role of observational learning and reinforcement in childhood socialization (Bandura, 1989). The acquisition of internal health values and overt health behavior determined by parental role models is well documented in the child health behavior literature. Parents who behave in health-enhancing or health-destructive ways are teaching these behaviors to their children. Children may learn and adopt similar behavior strategies by imitating the health-related behavior of their caregivers (Garralda, 2000).

Research suggests that modeling of health behavior is the most effective technique for socializing children's health behavior (Garralda, 2000; Lau et al., 1990). The strongest support for the modeling effects of parents on children's health behavior comes from U.S. and British studies of the relations between parents' and children's smoking. These studies suggest that parents who smoke strongly increase the chances that their child will smoke; conversely, parents who do not smoke are equally if not more likely to have a child who does not smoke (Doherty & Allen, 1994; Bauman, Ennett, Pemberton, & Foshee, 2001; Fearnow, Chassin, Presson, & Sherman, 1998; Murray, Kiryluk, & Swan, 1985). However, these relations may be more complex than they first appear. Fearnow and colleagues studied almost 1,000 families with a child aged 5–14 years (Fearnow et al., 1998). Two determinants of parents' smoking behaviors – (1) how much a parent discourages, talks about, and monitors child smoking and (2) parental permissiveness about the child smoking at home – were significant in affecting children's smoking behavior. These results suggest that the value parents placed on their child's not smoking was predictive of these parent behaviors, but not as much as when parents had less negative beliefs about smoking or when parents were highly stressed. These findings suggest possible mediating factors in the relations among parent and child cigarette smoking. These results are also consistent in related studies that examine the impact of mediating factors on the relations between parent and adult alcohol use. For example, Brody and his colleagues (Brody, Flor, Hollett-Wright, McCoy, & Donovan, 1999) found that children's norms about alcohol use are multiply determined, and that these determinants include child temperament, parent–child relationship quality, and the interactions between these constructs. Specifically, children's alcohol use norms deviated from the standard of abstinence as their parents' norms did, but this association was moderated by child temperament and parent–child relationship quality. For children with less supportive and communicative relationships with their parents, as maternal alcohol use standards moved away from abstinence, children were more likely to endorse the norm of youth alcohol use. In contrast, for children who had more supportive and communicative relationships with their parents, no relationship existed between mothers' and children's alcohol use norms. Children with temperaments that placed them more at risk for liberal alcohol use norms demonstrated more liberal standards if their fathers' norms for alcohol use were inconsistent with abstinence and if the father–child relationship was less supportive and communicative. However, the alcohol use norms of temperamentally at-risk youths whose relationships with their fathers were more supportive and communicative did not move away from abstinence even when their fathers did not endorse the abstinence norm.

Other examples of health behavior that appear to be taught to children at least partially by parental modeling in studies of Euro-American children include use of seat belts in a moving car (Lau et al., 1990), use of medications (Ranelli et al., 2000), eating behavior (Dielman et al., 1982; Lau et al., 1990), exercise (Lau et al., 1990; Sallis et al., 1992), alcohol use (Lau et al., 1990), type A behavior patterns (Forgays, 1992), and reporting symptom of illness (Garralda, 2000).

Research with non-Euro-American samples on parental modeling of health behavior as a factor in children's health socialization is somewhat consistent with these findings. In studies of mothers' socialization of Latino children's eating habits, Olvera-Ezzell et al. (1990) found that whereas mothers did report using modeling to influence their children's mealtime behavior, this technique was used much less often than other techniques such as threats, bribes, punishments, and nondirective methods such as making suggestions, asking questions, and offering choices. Thus, although modeling appears to be a significant mechanism for understanding the relations between parents' and children's health behavior, cultural differences in maternal health socialization strategies appear to be present.

Investigators have begun to examine the role of modeling and reinforcement in childhood health socialization more closely (Bennett, Huntsman, & Lilley, 2000). Dunn-Greier and colleagues (Dunn-Greier, McGarth, Rourke, Latter, & D'Astous, 1986) found that adolescents who do not cope well with chronic pain, in comparison to those who do, have mothers who are more likely to demonstrate behavior that discourages adolescents' efforts to cope with an exercise task. Others have found that mothers who maintain positive environments for their children's pain, and create opportunities for their children to observe others in pain, have children who report more pain (Broome, Richtsmeier, Maikler, & Alexander, 1986; Rickard, 1988; Robinson, Alverez, & Dodge, 1990). Still other researchers suggest a parental basis for children's sick role behavior. Mechanic (1965) studied 350 fourth- through eighth-grade children and their mothers in order to investigate how children's health-related behaviors develop. Results indicated moderate relations between the extent to which mothers were attentive to their own illness symptoms and children's illness behavior, with only 31% of mothers being high reporters of their own symptoms and high reporters of their children's symptoms. However, in general, mothers tend to be more concerned and responsive with respect to their children's health than their own health. Although a very weak relation was found between mothers' attentiveness to symptoms and children's attentiveness to symptoms, a stronger relation was found between mothers' inclination to go to a doctor when they felt ill and their tendency to take their children to a doctor when the children felt ill (41% of the mothers in the study reported both little inclination to go to a doctor when they were ill and little inclination to take their children to a doctor when the children were ill). Although Mechanic utilized analytical methods that greatly limited the number of explanatory variables that could be considered simultaneously, this was a landmark study. Mechanic was able to demonstrate definite, although at times weak, mother–child relations in health attitudes and behaviors. This study became even more important when Mechanic conducted a follow-up investigation (Mechanic, 1979) in an attempt to examine the stability of the children's original responses. Although the follow-up assessment items were not entirely comparable to the earlier items, the results indicated some minor relations across the time points in health attitudes and behaviors. Young adults with fewer symptoms remembered their parents as concerned with the teaching of self-care and the promotion of positive health habits. The mothers of children who grew up to have fewer physical symptoms were positively oriented toward health rather than concerned with seeking medical attention for their children's minor illnesses.

Several researchers have studied the influence of parents' physical activity levels on children's physical activity levels. Children's physical activity levels have been an important focus of the research on the effect of parents' behavior on children's health because it is a very significant health-related behavioral factor with regard to chronic disease prevention (e.g., heart disease, diabetes) and health promotion. Moreover, childhood obesity, which is directly related to children's activity levels, has serious implications for children's physical and psychological health (Davison & Birch, 2001).

Adult physical activity is notoriously hard to increase with health promotion programs. A better understanding of the determinants of children's physical activity should permit the development of better prevention and intervention programs designed to increase both children's and adults' physical activity levels. Many studies have found a positive relation between parents' and children's physical activity levels (Lindquist, Reynolds, & Goran, 1999; Perusse, Tremblay, LeBlanc, & Bouchard, 1989; Sallis, Patrick, Frank, & Pratt, 2000; Sallis, Patterson, Buono, Atkins, & Nader, 1988). For example, in a study of 4- to 7-year-old children and their parents, Moore and her colleagues (Moore et al., 1991) monitored parents' and children's physical activity with a mechanical device for an average of more than 10 hours per day for about 9 days each over the course of a year. Children of active mothers were twice as likely to be active as children of inactive mothers, and children of active fathers were almost four times as likely to be active as children of inactive fathers. When both parents were active, children were almost six times as likely to be active as children of two inactive parents. Parents' modeling of physical activity, shared activities by family members, and the support of active parents of their participation in active activities are possible explanations of these findings, although genetically transmitted factors may also predispose children to increased levels of physical activity. However, although these studies suggest the importance of parental modeling and reinforcement on children's physical activity behavior, a minority of studies suggest that we have much more to learn about the ways in which parents socialize this aspect of children's health behavior (Godin & Shephard, 1986). For example, Sallis and his colleagues examined the role of parents in children's physical activity (Sallis et al., 1992). In a prospective study of almost 300 fourth-grade children and their parents, these researchers found that parents had only very limited influence on their children's physical activity. Parents' own physical activity, which was assumed to be modeling, and parents' encouragement of their children to be active were not at all related to their children's level of physical activity. Further research is necessary to better specify the nature of parents' influence, via modeling and reinforcement, on children's physical activity behavior.

Walker and Zeman (1992), in a study of parents' responses to their children's illness behavior, found that mothers encourage their children's illness behavior more than fathers. They also found that mothers reportedly encouraged illness behavior related to gastrointestinal symptoms more than cold symptoms. These studies underscore the effectiveness of parental modeling and reinforcement of children's health behavior.

A significant area of research related to parental modeling and reinforcement effects on children's health behavior is concerned with parental influences on children's coping with medical procedures. Researchers in this area have explored a variety of issues related to parental competence in facilitating children's health treatment, including parental influences on children's fear and coping during inpatient and outpatient pediatric medical visits (Melamed, 1998; Rushforth, 1999). These studies suggest that a variety of behaviors, including parental use of distraction and low rates of ignoring, are associated with less child distress and increased child prosocial behavior (Stephens, Barkey, & Hall, 1999). Several specific maternal behaviors appear to be related to the extent of child distress during these procedures, including maternal agitation and reassurance. Other studies have focused exclusively on mothers' behavior during their children's immunizations and help us understand the direction-of-effects issue in these relations. Cohen and colleagues (Cohen, Manimala, & Blount, 2000) examined the relations among parents' reports of their usual behaviors during their children's immunizations, their observed behavior coded from videotapes, and children's coping and distress during immunization procedures. Results suggest that mothers overestimated the quantity of their soothing behaviors and that no relation existed between mothers' reports of the behavior and their actual behavior during their children's immunization procedures. Furthermore, mothers' reports of their behavior were unrelated to their children's distress or coping. However, parents' behaviors were significantly related to children's distress, with parental agitation negatively related and parental soothing positively related to children's coping. These findings suggest that mothers' behavior (in contrast to mothers' reports of their own behavior) should be used to evaluate the necessity for training in how to help children cope with aversive medical procedures like immunizations.

Bush and her colleagues (Bush, Young, & Radecki-Bush, 1998) have studied maternal influences on children's fear and coping during outpatient pediatric medical visits. These studies suggest that a variety of behaviors, including parental use of distraction and low rates of ignoring, are associated with lower child distress and more child prosocial behavior. Mothers' self-reports of positive reinforcement were associated with better child adjustment, and poorer child adjustment was related to punishment. Several maternal behaviors were related to child distress during these procedures, including maternal agitation and reassurance. Another study focused exclusively on mothers' behavior during their children's immunizations (Broome & Endsley, 1989). The results of this study shed some light on the direction-of-effects issue in these relations. Mothers' anxiety was self-reported, and children's anxiety was measured by the mothers immediately preceding the immunizations. Mothers' and children's behaviors were assessed during the actual immunizations. These observations revealed that most mothers reacted positively during the immunizations, reassuring their children with such statements as "You're doing really well" and "It's almost over!" Mothers' ratings of their own anxiety before the immunizations were not related to their behavior during the immunizations or to their children's behavior. However, mothers' ratings of their children's anxiety were positively related to their ratings of their own anxiety, and mothers' ratings of their children's anxiety were related to the children's behavior during their immunizations; children whose mothers rated them as more anxious were far more distressed and less cooperative during the immunizations. These findings suggest that mothers anticipate their children's anxiety about these procedures and become anxious themselves.

Several researchers have focused on the question of whether parents' presence during their children's minor medical procedures is really helpful. There are two views on this issue. The first view is that children demonstrate more negativity when their parents are present during anxiety-producing medical procedures than when they are absent. Researchers who support this position cite operant conditioning theory, which suggests that most children have a history of having their mother comfort them when they display distress and she eliminates aversive stimuli for them. Therefore, the mother acquires discriminative stimulus value for the child during aversive situations. In other words, the presence of the mother during an unpleasant medical procedure serves as a signal to the child that predicts a favorable outcome (e.g., comforting) if the child shows distress (e.g., crying) (Gonzalez et al., 1989; Stephens et al., 1999). For example, Gross and colleagues studied children between the ages of 4 and 10 who were having their blood drawn (Gross, Stern, Levin, Dale, & Wojnilower, 1983). Immediately before the blood test, children whose mothers were present cried more than children whose mothers were absent. The second view suggests that children are more emotionally aroused when their mothers are present, which accounts for their increased crying during the medical procedure. Support also exists for this hypothesis; Shaw and Routh (1982) found that children experiencing an aversive medical procedure are more likely to cry and fuss when their mothers are present. Although more research is needed to reconcile these contradictory findings, Gonzalez and his colleagues (1989) remind us that in studies of children's subjective reports of the effect of parental presence during aversive medical procedures, children overwhelmingly prefer their parents to be present. These authors suggest that

> having the parent present makes the child feel more secure and that separating a child from his or her parent for the purpose of administering a minor painful medical procedure is an unjustified practice. While it is true that a child may behave a bit worse if the parent is present, the importance of having the parent there must not be underestimated. In our opinion a child's wish to remain with the parent during painful procedures should be honored as long as the circumstances permit. (p. 461)

Other related questions concern whether parents want to be present during their children's medical procedures and whether medical personnel want parents to be there. A recent study addressed both of these questions. Bauchner and his colleagues observed 50 children (average age about 3 years) and their parents during each child's emergency room visit (Bauchner, Waring, & Vinci, 1991). Children were undergoing at least one of the following procedures: venipuncture or intravenous cannulation, bladder catheterization, or lumbar puncture. Sixty-two percent of the parents (31 of 50) chose to stay with their children during the procedure for a variety of reasons: They (1) thought their child wanted them to be in the room (90%), (2) wanted to know what the physician was doing to their child (77%), and (3) thought it would help to calm their child (81%). Only 43% reported that the medical personnel present asked them to stay with their child during the procedure. Of the 19 parents who did not stay with their children during the procedure, 42% said they would have liked to remain with their child, 26% stated that they did not want to be with their child, and 32% said that they did not know that they could have stayed with their child. Seven of the 19 parents who did not stay with their child reported that the physicians asked them to leave, although in four of these instances, the physicians denied this. Physicians did indicate that they thought parents should leave in 12 instances; 10 parents agreed. During 11 procedures, the physicians gave nonverbal cues, such as turning their backs on the parent or pulling the curtain behind them, that were interpreted to mean that the parent should leave. Physicians and nurses were asked whether they thought parents should stay with their children during these procedures. The majority of them responded that parents should be with their children during venipuncture (58%), but few believed that parents should be present during their children's lumbar puncture (14%). Of the medical personnel who felt that parents should not be present during these procedures, the reasons given included the following: (1) it makes the parents nervous or upset (93%), (2) the parents do not understand what is happening (60%), (3) it makes the physician nervous (46%), (4) it makes the child more upset (40%), or (5) the parents get in the way (40%). These results suggest relatively little agreement between parents and medical personnel about parental presence during unpleasant child medical procedures.

Is mothers' use of modeling as a health socialization strategy a cross-cultural phenomenon? Research suggests that Euro-American mothers are more likely than African American or Haitian mothers to report using modeling in dealing with their children during fear-inducing pediatric situations such as injections (Reyes, Routh, Jean-Gilles, & Sanfilippo, 1991). Melamed (1998), in an essay on maternal influences on children's coping with medical procedures, suggests that much more research in this area is needed to sort out the definition of parental competence in these situations and the developmental trajectories of parental influences on children's competence during medical events. Furthermore, research on the impact of parents' behavior during medical procedures has focused almost exclusively on the mother. Future research in this area should investigate both maternal and paternal behavior with respect to children's coping with medical procedures specifically and with illness generally.

Thus far, we have discussed the indirect ways in which parents' behavior affects children's health. Now we examine parents' efforts to influence children's health orientation through direct tutoring and training.

Parents' Establishment, Training, and Enforcement of Children's Health Behavior

The emergence of young children's ability to control and regulate their own health behavior is a very important aspect of parents' socialization of children's health behavior. Researchers who study childhood behavioral socialization believe that children's ability to self-regulate develops as a function of their emerging ability to engage in behavior that they understand to be approved of as a result of their caregivers' transmission of standards of behavior (Gralinski & Kopp, 1993). Research on childhood socialization has focused on a number of factors influencing the effectiveness of parental socialization of children, including parental factors that mediate its effectiveness (e.g., responsiveness, warmth, control) (Baumrind, 1978). Other research has examined the nature of parents' rules, as communicated to their children through the socialization process, and how these rules change developmentally. LeVine has posited that socialization is aimed first at protecting children and later at promoting family and cultural standards (LeVine, 1974). More recently, Gralinski and Kopp (1993), in a longitudinal study of mothers' rules for everyday standards of behavior, have demonstrated that mothers' earliest socialization efforts are focused on ensuring children's safety, and as children age (18–30 months), mothers shift their socialization attention to other issues including children's self-care. Finally, by age $3\frac{1}{2}$ years, mothers elaborate on previously established rules, and combine categories of rules about self-care and social norms (e.g., you must be dressed before you go out-doors). Other findings from this study suggest that safety rules are very im-portant to mothers. Interestingly, very young children's compliance with mothers' safety rules is highly advanced, in contrast to children's compli-ance with other categories of mothers' rules. These findings suggest the early and sustained salience of safety rules for both parents and children, and highlight the importance of further research on the description of the developmental pathways associated with parents' socialization of health and safety rules. However, other researchers question the extent of par-ents' attempts to socialize children's injury prevention behavior. Peterson and her colleagues (Peterson, Bartelstone, Kern, & Gillies, 1995) studied the ways in which mothers provide lectures and other remediative ac-tions following children's injuries. From an examination of written and oral children's and mothers' reports of over 1,000 injuries in 8-year-old children, these investigators found that parental use of such interventions as environmental change, discipline, or restriction of children's activity following childhood injury occurred in less than 3% of the child injuries studied, despite the fact that mothers were aware of over 92% of the in-juries. Most of the remediative behavior in which the parents did engage consisted of lectures about safety; however, most of the lectures were not even recognized by the children as such. These findings suggest that additional efforts are needed to teach parents to identify children's risky behavior and risky environmental situations, and how and when to use routine injury preventive intervention.

With respect to the impact of parents' direct training and enforce-ment of children's health behavior, research suggests that parents ex-plicitly attempt to train their children in health behavior, and that this is an important channel through which parents socialize their children's behavior (Lau et al., 1990). Moreover, this training begins very early. In the United States, parents introduce normative standards of cleanli-ness to their 2-year-old children (Kagan, 1982). Wilkinson (1988) believes that this timing is dependent on the child's sense of self, so that "the child's deviations from his sense of what is constant can be noted, disorder is dis-tinguished from order and unclean discriminated from clean" (p. 134) (see Douglas, 1966).

Parental training of children's health behavior is not always successful, and in fact may produce negative effects. For example, Johnson, Birch, and McPhee (1991) found that mothers who attempt to protect their children from obesity may create children who do not know how to stop eating when they have had enough. Their study of 77 children aged 3 to 5 years found that those with the most body fat had the most controlling mothers concerning the amount of food eaten. The more control the mother reported using to manage her child's eating behavior, the less food self-regulation the child demonstrated. In contrast, children whose mothers allowed them to be spontaneous about food (e.g., eating when they were hungry and not forced to finish all the food given them) displayed a natural instinct for regulating their own food intake. These findings appear to hold cross-culturally as well. In a Japanese study, the mothers of young adolescent girls were found, as reported by the mothers and daughters, to contribute to their daughters' eating disorder tendencies through control and monitoring (Mukai, Crago, & Shisslak, 1994). Another study focused on the role of parents in promoting children's physical activity found that parental encouragements to be active played no role in fourth graders' activity level (Sallis et al., 1992).

Although much more research is needed to clarify the most effective ways for parents to train their children about health, the results of another study may be helpful. Juanillo and Scherer (1991) studied the role of family communication about health in family health behaviors, knowledge, and attitudes. Findings suggested that talking with family members about the relation between diet and exercise and heart disease was positively related to family members' knowledge about the relation between these factors and health and negatively related to fat consumption. Although only husbands' and wives' health communication was studied, these results suggest a sound basis for the effect of family members' informational exchange on health behavior issues and lend support to the importance of parents' health-related teaching for childhood health socialization.

Beyond the Individual Level of Analysis: The Family as a Health Socialization Unit

The preceding studies focus on individual levels of analysis; parents have usually been represented by mothers, and in only a few cases by both fathers and mothers. However, it is important to consider a broader range of effects within the family as well as the family itself as a unit of analysis when considering parental influences on children's health orientation. What are the consequences of identifying family-level influences on children's promotion of health? What advantage does this approach give us in contrast to considering children's health at the individual level (e.g., the child affecting her or his own health or the mother's attitudes and behavior as determinants of the child's health)?

First, our current models of health suggest that health status is the result of an interaction of biological, social, and environmental factors. An understanding of the social and environmental contexts in which children exist is a critical ingredient of any model of childhood health. The family is the major component of young children's social and environmental contexts, and therefore knowledge of the role that the family plays in determining childhood health is necessary. Moreover, familial influence on children's health must be examined from multiple perspectives.

The role of individual family members in affecting children's health is obviously very important. For example, studies indicate that mothers play a pivotal role in determining the health of their children. Mothers have assumed a dominant role in performing health-related activities for all family members, particularly young children (Carpenter, 1990). Studies suggest that although fathers are making modest gains in participating in child care in general (Parke, 2000), mothers continue to be assigned child health care responsibilities in the division of household labor. Several studies suggest that a substantial cause of women's work absenteeism is caregiving for ill children (e.g., Carpenter, 1990), with women reporting about three times as many work hours lost as men for this task. Mothers have been found to take greater responsibility for family health (Hibbard & Pope, 1993). In a study of the extent to which members of almost 700 families with children had similar and interrelated health behavior, Schor, Starfield, Stidley, and Hankin (1987) found that although overall rates of use of health services by children were affected by the utilization rates of both parents, the effect of the mother was 2.3 times that of the father, and only mothers' utilization rates significantly influenced children's rates of visits for non-illness care.

Other studies suggest that women play a predominant role in establishing the health behavior of their children, making decisions concerning health services utilization, delivering children for pediatric care, and providing home nursing care for ill children (Carpenter, 1990). Mothers appear to perform most of the needs assessment and access of formal medical services for children, and in addition usually deliver children for these services. In many families, the decision about whether to declare a child sufficiently ill to stay home from day care or school and to need medical services is left to the mother (Dallas, Wilson, & Salgado, 2000). Carpenter (1990, p. 1214) eloquently suggests that "Women are the principal brokers or arrangers of health services for their children.... The assignment of family health responsibilities to the female in her role as ... mother ... is deeply rooted in cultural norms."

Is there a family-level assessment of health attitudes, health behavior, or health outcome that predicts children's health attitudes, health behavior, or health outcome better than any individual family member's predictors? In our own work (Tinsley, Markey, Ericksen, Kwasman, & Ortiz, 2002) on parental socialization of children's health beliefs and behaviors in Mexican American families, health constructs concerned with eating and exercise beliefs and behaviors, and their relations to obesity, are examined within the context of acculturative status. The health beliefs of 9- to 11-year-old fourth-grade Mexican American children and their parents are significant predictors of the child's, mother's, and father's body mass index. Health behaviors, however, significantly predict body mass index only for the mothers in our study. Path analyses of these data suggest that a best-fit model includes information from both mothers and fathers in the prediction of their children's body mass index.

Campbell (1975), in a discussion of the validity of intergenerational predictors of illness concepts, suggested that a combination of paternal and maternal influences would probably predict concordance between parents and children rather than the sole use of maternal influence. However, more than 25 years later, research is still needed to clarify these relations. A study of children who come from families in which there is a parent with somatization disorder (i.e., having physical symptoms out of proportion to demonstrable physical disease) suggested that having a somatizing parent was highly predictive of child somatization (Livingston, Witt, & Smith, 1995). Children with somatization disorder were found to visit the emergency room with greater than normal frequency, and to exhibit more suicidal behavior and more disability. Additionally, children in families with an adult with severe somatization disorder had almost 12 times the number of emergency room visits and missed almost 9 times as much school as children in families with a less severely affected somatizing adult. These data demonstrate that family patterns of medical care utilization are influenced by family definitions of illness, as well as frequency of disease.

Another example of family members' influence on children's health comes from a study of preschool children's ability to identify alcohol by odor as a function of fathers' and mothers' alcohol consumption (Noll, Zucker, & Greenberg, 1990). Results demonstrated that very young children's (31 to 69 months old) success in identifying alcoholic beverages by smell was positively related to paternal and maternal alcohol usage. This study suggests that the home is the context in which children learn about health-related risk behaviors such as drinking alcohol. It also demonstrates that young children's knowledge of this risky health behavior must be obtained from sources other than television (since odors are not part of television programming), despite the proliferation of television portrayals of alcohol consumption (Austin & Johnson, 1997).

In a consideration of family determinants of health behavior (for both adults and children), Sallis, Nader, and their colleagues conducted a series of studies suggesting that one major mechanism for family influence on health is an examination of the similarities and differences in health variables across family members (Broyles, Nader, Sallis, & Frank-Spohrer, 1996; Elder et al., 1998; McKenzie, Nader, Strikmiller, & Yang, 1996; Nader, Sellers, Johnson, & Perry, 1996; Perry et al., 1997). For example, with health variables related to cardiovascular disease, there are statistically significant correlations among parent–child, sibling–sibling, and spouse–spouse blood pressures. Although genetic influences account for part of the variance in at least parent–child and sibling–sibling blood pressure similarities, this is not the case for spouse–spouse blood pressures. Therefore, not all the variance is explained genetically. Similar family patterns are found with serum cholesterol, lipoproteins, and body fat (obesity). It is apparent that there are environmental family influences on health behavior and risk. Sallis and Nader and their colleagues (Broyles et al., 1996; Elder et al., 1998; McKenzie et al., 1996; Nader et al., 1996; Perry et al., 1997) discussed three such possible influences: smoking, diet, and exercise. There is a great deal of evidence that smoking habits (Scheer, Borden, & Donnermeyer, 2000), health-related dietary habits, and physical activity habits (Sallis et al., 2000) aggregate within families. However, many of the studies that provide this evidence are limited in terms of their attention to family structure, demographic variables, and the explication of comparative strengths and interactions of various influences (Sallis et al., 2000). These are empirical questions that must be answered in order to fully understand the role of the family in determining children's health attitudes and behavior. The influence of ethnicity and culture on parents' promotion of children's health are examples of such variables requiring additional empirical examination.

Epidemiological studies suggest an overrepresentation of health problems in minority children living in the United States compared to the population of U.S. children at large. Among the most vulnerable and dependent members of any community, children reflect the conditions of their communities within the larger societal context. As a result, the health status of ethnic children in the United States mirrors and magnifies that of their families and neighborhoods, as well as the effectiveness of the formal and informal institutional structures entrusted to meet their health needs (Halfon, Newacheck, Hughes, & Brindis, 1998; Harkness & Keefer, 2000). Children reared in the plethora of culturally diverse families in the United States are exposed to many conflicting health values and orientations, and these shift over time as a function of such changing phenomena as parental and family acculturation, education, geographic dispersion, and household structure and size. For many children reared in the United States, poverty is the main enemy of optimal health and ranks among the most significant factors affecting children's health.

Work on socialization patterns in minority families suggests that no single pattern characterizes a particular ethnic group; instead, parents adapt their socialization practices in response to sociocultural values (Julian, McKenry, & McKelvey, 1991). Studies have identified significant variation associated with ethnicity in attitudes about parenting, childrearing goals, types of parenting behaviors, and amount of parental involvement. Culture and ethnicity are also fundamental to health beliefs and behavior, and must be included in relevant theories and empirical investigations of parents' health promotion on behalf of their children (Landrine, Klonoff, Campbell, & Reina-Patton, 2000). However, to date, with few exceptions, studies have failed to examine systematically cultural and ethnic influences on parents' health promotion efforts.

One exception is a study by Lees and Tinsley (2000). Thirty-eight Mexican-origin preschool children and their mothers and 44 Euro-American children and their mothers participated in an investigation of patterns of maternal socialization of children's preventive health behaviors. Mothers reported their parenting practices by completing questionnaires about their health beliefs, parenting beliefs, and parenting practices. Children's handwashing, healthy food selection, and danger avoidance were independently reported by the children's preschool teachers. Patterns of parent beliefs and parenting practices that contributed to children's autonomous performance of healthy and safe behavior, as reported independently by the children's teachers, were identified. The patterns of the Mexican-origin mothers were unique and were not similarly associated with the successful maternal health socialization of the Euro-American preschoolers. Findings also demonstrated some domain specificity of Mexican-origin maternal socialization practices, whereby specific parenting strategies were differentially related to the three categories of child health behavior: handwashing, healthy food selection, and danger avoidance. Theoretically, the findings of this study provide information about unique family processes associated with ethnicity that impact the parenting behavior of Mexican-origin mothers and that serve to socialize their young children's health and safety.

Conclusions

Parents unquestionably aim to promote their children's health, but there are many obstacles to successful socialization of children's health and well-being. New models of child health care that incorporate both biological and experiential components of children's health have facilitated attempts to overcome these obstacles. Research suggests that parents' modeling of health attitudes and behaviors has the potential to influence those of their children, resulting in greater child well-being. Particular parenting behaviors (e.g., positive reinforcement) have also been linked to children's development of adaptive health behaviors. Furthermore, parents play an important role in helping children cope with illness and medical treatments.

5

Parents' Promotion of Their Children's Sexual Health

Children's Education about Sexuality

One important health-related area in which parents explicitly train children is sexuality (Geasler, Dannison, & Edlund, 1995; Klein & Gordon, 1992; Meschke, Zweig, Barber, & Eccles, 2000; Miller, Forehand, & Kotchick, 1999, 2000). Empirical evidence demonstrates that open, supportive family communication patterns foster positive parent–child relationships and encourages adolescents to internalize the values and mores embedded in their parents' messages (Newcomer & Udry, 1985; Whitaker & Miller, 2000). Many youth report interest in having open discussions with their parents regarding sexuality and HIV (Krauss, 1997). Furthermore, research has illuminated the strong links among family communication about sexuality, parent–child relationship quality, and adolescents' risky behavior (Baldwin & Baranowski, 1990; Forehand & Kotchick, 1996). Studies have consistently documented the role of parent–child communication about sex in adolescents' responsible sexual behavior and deterrence of early sexual activity (Crosby et al., 2000; DiIorio, Kelley, & Hockenberry-Eaton, 1999; Howard & McCabe, 1992; Kotchick, Shaffer, & Forehand, 2001; Murry, 1996; Scott-Jones & Turner, 1990), and more consistent condom use (Kotchik et al., 2001; Whitaker & Miller, 2000).

The timing of parent–adolescent sexual communication appears to be significant. Inner-city African American and Hispanic adolescents whose mothers discussed condom use with them before they became sexually active were three times more likely to use condoms the first time they had sex and three times more likely to use condoms consistently

57

(Miller, Kotchick, Dorsey, Forehand, & Ham, 2001). When parent–child communication about sex occurs after adolescents' sexual debut, research suggests that parents are most effective when tailoring their sex education messages according to the sexual experience of their children (i.e., whether adolescents are in monogamous relationships or are engaging in sexual activity with multiple partners) (Shrier, 2001).

Parent–child communication may influence adolescents' sexual values and perceptions of sexual norms (DiIorio et al., 1999), leading to the development of sexual values that are more conservative and similar to those of their parents. Parents may also serve as a buffer against peer pressure to engage in sexual activity by providing continual reinforcement of norms and beliefs (Santelli, DiClemente, Miller, & Kirby, 1999; Whitaker & Miller, 2000). Inner-city adolescent girls who discussed with their parents when they should have sex were less influenced by whether they thought their friends had initiated sexual activity early or later than were those who had not had such a discussion with their parents (Whitaker & Miller, 2000).

What do parents and children talk about when they discuss sex? Rosenthal and Feldman, among other researchers, in two studies, suggest that parent–adolescent conversations about sex are focused more on the less intimate and personal issues of sexuality, including developmental change (e.g., menstruation onset). Much less frequent are conversations concerned with such topics as masturbation, nocturnal emissions, access to contraceptives, orgasm, or sexual decision making (Baldwin & Baranowski, 1990; Feldman & Rosenthal, 2000; Rosenthal & Feldman, 1999).

What factors influence the extent to which parents engage in conversations with their children about sex? Parents expect to train children explicitly about sex (Simanski, 1998). However, despite the fact that parents appear to be willing to teach their children about sexuality (Berne, Patton, Milton, & Hunt, 2000), parents have beliefs discrepant from those of their children concerning their perceived extent to which they talk to their children about sex and the sexual topics covered (Jaccard, Dittus, & Gordon, 1998; King & Lorusso, 1997; Rosenthal & Feldman, 1999). Parents may be reluctant to discuss sexual matters with their children and adolescents because of discomfort in discussing sexual topics in general; personal, moral, or religious beliefs that adolescent premarital sex is wrong; concerns that discussing sexuality and safe sex may promote adolescent sexual activity; lack of knowledge regarding the risks of various behaviors; and lack of communication skills (Jaccard, Dittus, & Gordon, 2000).

One study has examined the role of two parental social cognitive variables in determining parents' engagement with their children about sexuality. DiIorio and colleagues (DiIorio et al., 2000) found that mothers who expressed greater self-efficacy and more favorable outcome expectancies in talking to their children about sex were more likely to have these conversations. Similarly, Raffaelli and her colleagues (Raffaelli, Bogenschneider, & Flood, 1998) found that parents' beliefs about the sexual behavior of their child and his or her peers were related to their adolescents' reports of sexual communication. For mothers, believing that their adolescent's friends were sexually active was related to the extent of engaging in discussions with their children about the legitimacy of adolescent sexual behavior. For fathers, the belief that other adolescents are engaging in sexual behavior was related to having discussions with their youths about sexually transmitted diseases (STDs), acquired immune deficiency syndrome (AIDS), and contraceptives. Mothers with concerns about their children's sexuality and fathers who believe that adolescent sex is acceptable or inevitable had discussions about STDs and AIDS with their youths. These authors suggest that parents who are more concerned about sexuality communicate more directly than do parents who are less concerned.

As the preceding review suggests, there are mother–father differences in various aspects of parents' communication about sex and sexuality with adolescents. Mothers and fathers demonstrate different styles in discussions of sex. Studies suggest that mothers, more than fathers, tend to (1) recognize and accept adolescents' opinions about sex-related topics, (2) initiate and engage in these conversations, and (3) receive adolescents' self-disclosures about sex (Feldman & Rosenthal, 2000; Noller & Callan, 1990). Overall, communication about these topics appears to be the province of mothers, particularly with daughters (Feldman & Rosenthal, 2000). Fathers, compared to mothers, are more likely to discuss sexual topics with sons (DiIorio et al., 1999). When fathers do have these conversations, they tend to focus on the least intense and intimate aspects of these topics (Hepburn, 1983). Both mothers and fathers are reported by their adolescents to be uncomfortable during these discussions, which have been characterized, over several studies, as indirect, involving more dominance and unilateral power assertion, less mutuality, and less turn-taking than during conversations about more benign topics. Adolescents are characterized as equally discomfited by these conversations, and their behavior is described as involving more contempt, less honesty, and more avoidance than they display in conversations with their parents about other topics (Rosenthal & Feldman, 1999; Kahlbaugh, Lefkowitz, Valdez, & Sigman, 1997; Lefkowitz, Kahlbaugh, & Sigman, 1996; Rosenthal & Feldman, 2000; Yowell, 1997).

Several other studies have demonstrated cultural differences in the way families talk to their children about sex, human immunodeficiency syndrome (HIV), and AIDS (Crawford, Thomas, & Zoller, 1993). Baumeister, Flores, and Marin (1995) found that Hispanic adolescents report less communication with their parents about sexuality than do non-Hispanic adolescents. In an investigation of a specific subgroup of Euro-American, Hispanic, and African American parents and children (i.e., those living in transitional living shelters for the homeless), parents were interviewed about their HIV/AIDS knowledge, attitudes, and communication with their children. Results indicated that (1) Euro-American and African American parents discussed HIV/AIDS more often with their children than did Hispanic parents; (2) more well-educated parents were more knowledgeable about and reported greater frequency of parent–child communication about sex and HIV than did those with less education; and (3) African American mothers were significantly less likely to perceive themselves at risk for HIV infection than were Euro-American mothers (Crawford et al., 1993). In light of epidemiological evidence demonstrating that African Americans and Hispanics are at greater risk of HIV infection than other groups, and at the same time perceive a lower risk and talk less with their children about it, these findings suggest further critical barriers to HIV prevention in those families.

Children's own reports of family communication about sex and HIV/AIDS produce similar findings. A sample of 207 fifth graders, balanced for ethnicity (one-half African American and one-half Euro-American) and gender, were more likely to report that their parents had not discussed HIV/AIDS with them if they were African American or had parents with lower education or income. This agrees with a Centers for Disease Control (CDC) report on the characteristics of parents who discuss HIV/AIDS with their children (CDC, 1991), which demonstrates that Hispanic parents and parents living in large metropolitan areas (which incorporate large population groups of low-socioeconomic status African American families) also discuss HIV/AIDS less often with their children. Thus, low-income and/or African American and Hispanic families, who are at greater risk for new HIV infection than are Euro-Americans and those of higher socioeconomic status, are engaging in less, and/or less accurate, parent–child communication about HIV/AIDS. This may be due to discomfort about discussing sensitive issues such as sex, a greater focus on more proximal problems due to poverty and/or neighborhood dangers, or lack of understanding or perception of the level of risk they and their children incur. More research on the relations of these demographic variables and cause(s) of this lack of communication about HIV/AIDS is necessary.

Examinations of the sources of sexual information for Euro-American and Hispanic adolescents demonstrate ethnic differences in parental discussions about adolescent sexual behavior. For example, Gomez and Marin (1996) report that Hispanic women do not commonly talk about sex, AIDS, or condoms because it can be regarded as disrespectful, distasteful, or indicative of promiscuity in the Hispanic culture. Euro-American adolescent males appear more likely to report getting information about sex from their parents than do Hispanic adolescent males (Moran & Corley, 1991). Results of this study also indicate that sex education has a greater influence on condom use among Hispanic compared to Euro-American male adolescents and that young Hispanic males living in traditional homes do not ask questions about sex out of respect for their elders, suggesting that when sexual communication with parents is not available, adolescents access information elsewhere. However, a study by Pillado, Romo, and Sigman (2000) suggests that the acculturation level may modify these patterns. In a further reminder of the importance of examining sources of intraethnic variance in studies of parent–child communication about sex, Pillado and her colleagues examined the range of topics discussed in Hispanic mother–child conversations about sexuality. Hispanic girls and their mothers were videotaped discussing dating and sexuality. Considerable variability was found among these dyads concerning sensitive sexual issues, especially dating, pregnancy, HIV, and other dangers associated with sexual behavior, as a function of language preference (Spanish, English). With a more international perspective with respect to assessment of youths' knowledge and attitudes about HIV and AIDS, as well as the sources of these attitudes and knowledge, 80% of Chinese adolescents have rarely or never discussed HIV/AIDS with their families (Davis, Noel, Chan, & Wing, 1998).

Other research suggests the importance of parents' continuing efforts to socialize their children about sexuality. Parent–child communication about sexuality appears to make a difference in youths' sexual risk-taking. Adolescents who report discussing a greater number of topics about sexuality with their mothers were less likely to have initiated sexual intercourse than other youths (DiIorio et al., 1999). Blum et al. (2000) examined relations among youths' perceptions of their mothers' approval of sexual activity and the timing of their first intercourse, utilizing data from a national survey of U.S. children in Grades 7 to 12. Results indicated that adolescents' perceptions of high maternal disapproval of sexual activity and high levels of maternal connectedness (measured by both adolescents' and mothers' reports) were each independently related to delay in first intercourse. Thirteen- to 19-year-old Hispanic girls reporting higher levels of parental communication about sex were less likely to be pregnant (Baumeister et al., 1995). In another investigation, adolescents who talked to parents about sex reported less sexual experience, fewer pregnancies, and more HIV prevention behavior, consisting primarily of condom use (Leland & Barth, 1993). A third study suggests that adolescents who perceived strong maternal disapproval of sexual activity and who were strongly connected to their mothers were most likely to delay their sexual intercourse debuts (Blum et al. 2000). These studies suggest that parent–adolescent communication about sexuality is positively related to similarities in sexual attitudes and values among parents and children, delayed sexual experience, use of condoms, and pregnancy prevention. However, the extent of these discussions about sex and other risk behaviors may be curtailed by culturally related values and expectations and by other psychosocial environmental factors. In general, parents and adolescents do not speak sufficiently about sexuality (Hutchinson & Cooney, 1998). As a result, adolescents overestimate maternal approval of their sexual behavior, and mothers underestimate the amount of sexual activity of their adolescents (Jaccard et al., 1998).

Parent–adolescent communication about sex appears to decrease HIV risk behaviors (Leland & Barth, 1993). Youth reporting parent–adolescent discussions about sex are more likely to delay sexual activity (Darling & Hicks, 1982). Mother–adolescent discussions regarding condom use prior to the first sexual intercourse increase the chances of condom use during the first and subsequent sexual encounters (Christopherson, Miller, & Norton, 1994; Miller, Levin, Whitaker, & Xu, 1998; Christ, Raszkat, & Dillon, 1998; Whitaker & Miller, 2000).

Cultural factors may influence parental communication about HIV/AIDS. Parents' and children's orientations toward illness and communication about illness are constrained by cultural factors that influence understanding of the illness and treatment, as well as their decisions about and compliance with medical recommendations. For example, in families with an asthmatic third to fifth grader whose parents' preferred language was Spanish, there was more parent–child communication than in other families (DuRant, Sanders, Jay, & Levinson, 1990). In these cases, however, the children were communicating more to parents and making suggestions about how to manage their asthma, rather than information flowing from parent to child. However, in a different cultural group, the Hmong, parents were the best communicators of their child's current and past functional abilities as long as translators were available (Meyers, 1992). These contrasting findings may reflect cultural differences in communication patterns and roles within the family. Thus, Euro-American parents may be more likely to discuss HIV/AIDS and prevention with their children and to encourage children's understanding and independent prevention efforts, while Hispanic parents may believe that they, the elders, should take care of their children's prevention – by protecting them from unsafe situations, for example.

Communication patterns vary greatly across ethnic groups, and this cultural diversity interacts with the gender and age of family members. The specific family members who are responsible for transmitting safety and/or health information to children also vary among cultural groups. Non-Hispanic white American families rely primarily on mothers for health and safety socialization (Tinsley, Markey, Erickson, Kwasman, & Ortiz, 2002). However, grandparents or other elders may be responsible for these activities in other cultural groups (Die-Trill, Bromberg, LaVally, & Portales, 1996), and these family members may not have access to accurate and/or appropriate information on these topics, or may not feel comfortable discussing sexual issues, for example, with children. Additionally, although mainstream American culture emphasizes communicating with ill children, sharing with them as much information about their illness as they are capable of understanding, other cultures do not encourage the discussion of illness and/or death with children (Die-Trill, Bromberg, LaVally, & Portales, 1996). Similarly, families with other ethnicities may not consider discussing a potentially fatal disease, HIV/AIDS, with their children for a variety of reasons (superstitious beliefs, attitudes about what children should and should not know, beliefs about children's readiness to understand, and so on) (Die-Trill et al., 1996). Thus, understanding the way cultural differences influence family management of chronic illness may shed some light on potential cross-cultural effects on family communication about one particular illness, HIV/AIDS, in terms of the influence of parenting practices and communication patterns.

Summary

The manner in which parents communicate expectations and set norms for their adolescents has a profound effect on youth behavior. The lack of open and comfortable discussions about sexuality, even in the most primary parent–child relationships, is a major concern for adolescent HIV risk (Institute of Medicine, 1997). Furthermore, cultural and ethnic variations in the manner in which these characteristics impact adolescent behavioral outcomes must be considered (Faryna & Morales, 2000). Communication about sex and drugs in adolescents' families affects preventive behavior and offers us important insights into how such families influence their children's drug use and sexual behavior. However, understanding how families communicate about HIV, and the cultural and societal modifiers of these effects, is critical to increase our understanding of these processes and their potential for use in HIV prevention (Perrino, Gonzalez-Soldevilla, Pantin, & Szapoczick, 2000). We now turn to a review of prior research on the extent and effects of parent–child communication on the risk of HIV to adolescents.

Intervention Studies

Most HIV prevention programs for youth have a group or classroom format addressed directly to adolescents. Although there is a considerable body of research documenting that parents and families can be effective facilitators of social and cultural learning, few programs have intervened beyond individual adolescents. Adopting a family perspective in adolescent HIV prevention efforts, however, is promising, as illustrated by recent studies. For example, Perrino and his colleagues (2000) designed and evaluated an intervention to increase parents' effectiveness in transmitting prevention information and techniques concerning HIV and other STDs to adolescents aged 10–13 years. Parents were taught what specific prevention information children need to know as they develop and are exposed to new and different risks. Results suggest that parent–adolescent communication about HIV, parents' and adolescents' knowledge about HIV, adolescents' intentions to use condoms during sexual intercourse, and their intention to avoid or reduce risky behaviors were all increased as a result of the intervention strategy (Krauss et al., 2000).

Can we teach families to communicate about sex and AIDS? Does improving family communication about HIV/AIDS improve children's knowledge of HIV and preventive behavior? Two investigations focusing on improving HIV/AIDS prevention behaviors by encouraging familial interaction and communication about AIDS have demonstrated some success (Crawford, Jason, Riordan, & Kaufman, 1990; Icard, Schilling, & El-Bassel, 1995). One investigation demonstrated possible ways that the amount and effectiveness of HIV/AIDS communication within African American families might be improved. African American families play a significant role in providing emotional support and socialization for family members, which in turn results in improved HIV preventive behavior in gay and bisexual men and intravenous (IV) drug users (Schilling, El-Bassel, Leeper, & Freeman, 1991; Leviton, Valdiserri, Lyter, & Callahan, 1990). The African American family is an effective source of AIDS information for family members, especially those who do not feel comfortable with standard outreach programs (Bowser & Wingood, 1992). Bowser employed the strengths of African American families, and the important function African American families have in health prevention, in designing their intervention. Parents in this study were exposed to either training about the biological and psychological aspects of sexuality and STDs or to the same training plus information about AIDS and training in communication and problem-solving skills. The intervention included discussions about cultural values affecting AIDS risk behaviors, the sexual relations of African Americans, and the effects of racism on African Americans' sexual behavior. African American parents, defined as any parent, grandparent, aunt, uncle, or unrelated adult responsible for a child, participated. Several aspects of the intervention were successful. First, the study demonstrated that African American parents are willing to enroll in and participate in a program about sexuality. Although participation in the enhanced program did not affect HIV/AIDS knowledge or participants' attitudes about talking to children about STDs and sex, the participants reported increased motivation to reduce or change their own high-risk behavior and reported that they were more comfortable talking about sex and HIV/AIDS to other adults after the intervention. Bowser and Wingood suggest that participation in this type of program may begin to overcome some of the stigma and cultural barriers that have prevented African Americans from participating in other HIV/AIDS prevention programs (Bowser, 1992). Investigations of the attitudes and beliefs of African American clergy toward sex education suggest an increasing desire among clergy and their congregations for health education programs in African American churches (Coyne-Beasley & Schoenbach, 2000). Thus, family sexual education relevant to the risk of HIV may be more likely, in the future, to be supplemented by education provided by such extrafamilial organizations as churches.

A second intervention study found that including parents of eighth graders of four different ethnicities (Euro-American, Hispanic, African American, and Asian) in media-based HIV/AIDS educational programs increased their knowledge and the frequency of discussions about HIV/AIDS with their children (Crawford et al., 1990). In this study, parents of eighth graders viewed a multimedia HIV/AIDS educational program consisting of televised elements and printed materials, including information on how to talk about AIDS as well as exercises to improve communication within the family. These parents (1) demonstrated increased knowledge on a posttest, (2) reported an increase in discussions about sex and HIV/AIDS with their children, and (3) reported viewing more AIDS prevention programming on television with their children than did control families (Crawford et al., 1990). These findings were particularly meaningful in light of the finding that most of the youth in the investigation (79%) reported engaging in behaviors that put them at high risk for HIV infection, including alcohol and drug use, unprotected sexual activity, and interactions with other high-risk individuals (e.g., friends who use IV drugs). These findings suggest that public programs such as these may encourage discussion of formerly taboo or uncomfortable subjects such as HIV/AIDS risk, drug use, and sexuality. Although the participants in this study were ethnically diverse (34% Euro-American, 20% Hispanic, 33% African American, and 5% Asian), the effectiveness of the intervention was not examined by ethnic group, limiting the ability to establish the potential interaction of ethnicity with intervention effectiveness.

Not all studies have demonstrated these effects of parental involvement on children's knowledge of HIV/AIDS or their related behavior. In one investigation, parental participation in a school-based HIV/AIDS educational program was not found to influence seventh-, eighth-, and ninth-grade students' behavioral intentions, knowledge, or attitudes over and above the influence of the educational program alone (Weeks, Levy, Gordon, & Handler, 1997). However, children whose parents participated in the program were significantly more likely to state that their parents' feelings about whether or not the children had sex were important. Moreover, participation in the treatment group (with or without parental involvement) enhanced children's knowledge and comfort in discussing sex and drugs with their parents; these effects appeared to be unrelated to the use of reported risk behaviors for the treatment group compared to the nontreatment controls. A limitation of the study was that, despite access to a large multiethnic sample, analyses by ethnicity were not offered. Other studies, as described previously, suggest that communication processes within families indicate significant cultural differences that might be demonstrated in analyses by ethnic group; for example, effects of parent involvement may differ in different ethnic groups, and further analyses of the Weeks et al. (1997) data on effects of ethnicity would increase the value of this investigation.

Summary

A few investigators have begun to examine the effects of parental communication on children's knowledge of HIV/AIDS and related behavior. They have found ethnic and/or cultural differences within families, with those groups at greatest risk for new HIV infection – African Americans, Hispanics, and low socioeconomic families – demonstrating less communication and less accurate knowledge. Additionally, some studies have demonstrated similarities in parent and child knowledge and attitudes about HIV/AIDS, suggesting intergenerational transmission, although changes in children's knowledge seems more closely related to developmental change in their understanding rather than to parental communication, at least at younger ages.

Increasingly, most physicians, educators, parents, and researchers agree that HIV/AIDS education is most productive and effective when begun when children are young, before the puberty and adolescence. Given that parents and adult caregivers are the primary socializers of children's healthy and preventive behaviors (Tinsley, 1992; Lees & Tinsley, 1998; Tinsley, Markey, Ericksen, Kwasman, & Ortiz, 2002). If children are to benefit from discussions of HIV transmission and prevention, their adult socializers must consider children's understanding of illness, disease and infection processes, and prevention behavior. However, despite the fact that parents appear to be willing to teach their children about sexuality (Wurtele, 1993), both parents and children believe that parents do not function well as sex educators (Klein & Gordon, 1992). In a survey of parents of children aged 3–11 years, Roberts and colleagues (Roberts, Kline, & Gagnon, 1978) found that most parents believe that one conversation about sexuality during children's development is enough. A variety of explanations have been offered for parents' inadequacies in delivering sex education, including fear that information about sexuality will give their children "ideas" (Klein & Gordon, 1992) and result in premature sexual behavior, discomfort in talking about sexuality (Koblinsky & Atkinson, 1982), and uncertainty about how to address sex education developmentally (Croft & Asmussen, 1992). For example, in a focus group study of parental concerns about sex education of fathers and mothers of preschool children, Geasler and her colleagues (1995) found several issues that worried parents. Parents were concerned about the age appropriateness of sex-related topics. One father remarked, "The thing that makes me feel uncomfortable is at what point do you really get down to details?" (p. 186). A mother asked, "What can they understand at a particular age? What should I be possibly looking for? Maybe if they aren't asking for...maybe I should be introducing things that aren't being asked. Am I going to wake up when they are teenagers and find out that I should have been addressing things that maybe didn't come up for one reason or another?" (p. 186).

Other parents were concerned about giving too much information. For example, one mother who had just given birth and was having a hard time explaining to her 4-year-old why she was bleeding said: "It's a struggle. It's a real struggle to know how far to go. I find myself trying to skirt around it because I'm afraid that one question is going to lead to another...and I'm afraid I'm going to give away too much" (p. 186). Another mother said about her 4-year-old daughter: "I want the innocence to last as long as I can. Just be a kid and have fun and don't think about this kind of stuff" (p. 186).

Many parents believe that our society pushes sexual information on children too early, which forces parents to address these issues earlier than they would prefer. One mother relates: "...We turn the TV on and my four-year-old is saying, 'Well, what's safe sex?' 'What's a condom?'" (p. 186). This same mother remembered watching an episode of the *Bill Cosby Show* with her daughter in which one character, Rudy, begins menstruating. She remarked: "I remember feeling a little bit of anger at that point that I'm being forced to be telling her something because we're watching some family television program, but in the long run, I'm kinda glad for it because it was an opportunity to start that conversation in a real nonfearful, nonpressuring type of environment" (p. 186).

Another issue concerning parents in educating their children about sex was the fear of communicating information to their children's friends and how their parents might react. One mother related the following story:

> My daughter and son bathe together a lot or we throw them in the shower together.... One of them had a friend over and my husband said to me, "Well, we'd better split everyone up." Well, everyone is

innocent and no one was thinking anything and I thought why should we draw attention to something that maybe there is no attention, but we just split everyone up. I didn't want this child to go home, and tell their folks. What are they going to say? (p. 186)

In an examination of parents' plans for sex education for their children, both mothers and fathers reported a wish to participate (Koblinsky & Atkinson, 1982). However, the roles that they play may be determined by other factors, such as social class. Hodson and Wampler (1988) found that although both middle-class and working-class parents felt comfortable discussing sexual topics with their children, working-class parents preferred that the mother take charge, whereas middle-class parents believed that both parents should be involved. Other studies of parent–child communication about sexuality suggest that mothers are the main agents of sexual socialization for boys and girls, but more so for girls (Nolin & Petersen, 1992). Mother–daughter communication appears to be more common than mother–son communication. These gender differences are most pronounced for discussions about sexuality focused on factual and moral topics, the types of communication most likely to transmit information and values (Nolin & Petersen, 1992). Fraley and her colleagues (Fraley, Nelson, Wolf, & Lozoff, 1991) asked 117 mothers of preschool children which words for genitals they used with their children. They found that preschool children were not likely to be given standard anatomical terms, although many children received "colorful and colloquial expressions" (p. 301). Girls were less likely than boys to have labels for their own genitals but were more likely to receive names for boys' genitals from their mothers.

One aspect of sexuality socialization that strongly concerns parents is the desire to improve on the sex education that they received as children. As the father of two young children commented, "My education, my parents. I don't know where they thought I got it because they didn't give it to me and I felt the same thing, you know. Hey, I'm going to do it differently with my child" (Geasler et al., 1995, p. 187). However, studies suggest that parents are not always adequate in conveying accurate sexual information to their children (Geasler et al., 1995). The reason may be somewhat related to a lack of parental knowledge about sexuality and about what is normal or acceptable at different developmental levels, but probably other factors are also involved. Geasler and her colleagues (1995) suggest that parental behavior related to sexuality often reflects the tension between parents' conflicting experiences of sexuality when they were young and their contemporary experience of sexuality with their children.

However, other research suggests the importance of parents' continuing efforts to socialize their children about sexuality. Parent–child communication about sexuality appears to make a difference; Fox and Inazu (1980) found that the frequency of mother–daughter communication about sexuality is linked to knowledge of birth control and responsible sexual behavior in adolescence. Adolescents whose parents communicated openly with them about sexuality in childhood report being much more comfortable discussing sexual topics with their parents and are more likely to make personal decisions about sexual behavior that reflect parental values (Brock & Jennings, 1993). In this era of AIDS, parental socialization of children's sexual knowledge has become a critical aspect of health socialization. Sigelman and her colleagues (Sigelman, Derenowski, Mullaney, & Siders, 1993) examined parents' propensity to discuss AIDS with their children in Grades 1–12. Although previous research suggests that children learn more about AIDS from television than from their parents (Fassler, McQueen, Duncan, & Copeland, 1990; McElreath & Roberts, 1992), findings indicated that the frequency of parent–child communication about AIDS was positively associated with children's knowledge about AIDS.

Evidence for the utility of explicit education about prevention comes from research addressing parents' role in teaching their children about sexual health. This and other health research is limited, however, in its focus on mothers' role in health promotion; additional research is needed to help understand the role of fathers. Moreover, the influence of entire families, conceptualized as a unit functioning in a greater cultural and ecological context, on children's health promotion needs further investigation.

6

Peers, Schools, and Children's Health

A comprehensive picture of the ways in which children are socialized about health must include sources of influence beyond the family such as peers and schools. These influences have traditionally been viewed as important in early and middle childhood, when children begin formal schooling. However, in light of recent changes in maternal employment patterns and the early use of day care for a large percentage of infants and toddlers, these extrafamilial socializing agents are potentially influential from an early age. According to recent U.S. government estimates, only a quarter of infants and toddlers are cared for by their parents; the remainder are cared for by relatives or in a day-care home or center (Clarke-Stewart, 1993). Clearly, peers and other adults have many opportunities to influence the development of children's health attitudes and behaviors.

Peers as Influences on Children's Health

In spite of the many studies concerning the role of peers as models or reinforcing agents among young children (Bandura, 1989; Hartup, 1996; Newcomb, Bukowski, & Pattee, 1993), there is little research on the impact of peers on young children's health attitudes and behavior. For the most part, outcomes of peer socialization have been explored in the domains of cognitive development, school achievement, and personal and social adjustment. To date, with the exception of studies on adolescent antisocial health-related behaviors (e.g., substance use, sexuality), which we will address later, none of these peer socialization processes has been empirically studied in the context of children's

health. In addition, research suggests that situational variables and individual differences among children (e.g., self-esteem, locus of control,
social status) impact on the effectiveness of these peer processes as
influences on children's behavior in general. Again, however, except
for the studies of adolescents' antisocial behavior, the impact of situational and individual difference factors as modifiers of peer influence
on children's health attitudes and behavior are virtually unexamined.
No studies have focused on the development of children's normative
health behavior, as influenced by peers. However, there is accumu-
lating evidence that early patterns of peer relations foreshadow later
behaviors such as risk-taking that are detrimental to children's health.
This work is particularly important since it may suggest ways of designing preventive and intervention programs to change adverse health
development.

Early Antecedents of Later Peer-Related Health Problems

Considerable evidence demonstrates that children can be identified as being at risk for later health-threatening behavior even in the
preschool period. In a New Zealand longitudinal study of 1,037 children
who were followed from age 3 to age 15, antisocial behavior at ages 11
and 15 was predicted by behavior problems in the preschool period, using both pediatrician and parent reports (White, Moffitt, Earls, Robins, &
Silva, 1990). However, not all children were correctly classified, and the
false positive prediction rate was high. Even more convincing evidence
suggests that children who are likely to be at risk in adolescence can
be identified in the earliest elementary school years. Vitaro, Tremblay,
and their colleagues have found that children who were rejected by their
peers in kindergarten not only remain rejected, but are more likely to develop social and academic problems in adolescence (Gagnon, Vitaro, &
Tremblay, 1992). Boys who are disruptive in Grade 1 are more likely to
be involved in delinquent behavior – high-risk and health-endangering
activities – at age 14 (Tremblay et al., 1992). Patterson and his colleagues
(Patterson, Capaldi, & Bank, 1991; Patterson, DeBaryshe, & Ramsey,
1989) have made a useful distinction between early and late starters.
Early starters are children who begin a pattern of deviant activity at a relatively young age (7–10 years), while *late starters* begin their risk-taking
activities only during preadolescence and adolescence. Follow-up studies
clearly indicate that early starters are more likely than late starters to be
at risk for a variety of health-related problems such as substance abuse

and antisocial aggressive behavior. Early starters are also more likely than late starters to be arrested as teens.

One of the major ways in which these rejected children maintain their at-risk behaviors is through self-selection into groups of peers with similar histories of deviant behavior and rejection (Cairns & Cairns, 1994; La Greca, Prinstein, & Fetter, 2001). Within these groups, rejected children maintain and refine patterns of behavior that are health-threatening, such as substance abuse, early sexual activity, and delinquent-aggressive behavior.

Do Peers Become a Hazard to Children's Health as Children Develop?

It is commonly assumed that as children age, they become more prone to engage in risky behavior as a result of the waning of parental control and the dominance of peer influence. However, empirical studies suggest that these assumptions may be, at best, oversimplifications (Brown, 1990). Research demonstrates, for example, that parents' influence on children's attitudes and behaviors, in comparison to that of peers, is much more substantial than has previously been acknowledged (Smetana, 1988). Moreover, peer influence on risky behavior has probably been overrated as a result of several methodological flaws in this area of research, including the fact that in most of these studies, child subjects report on their own as well as their friends' attitudes and behavior without independent validation (Hayes, 1987). Finally, evidence provided by Steinberg (1986) suggests that the relation between parent and peer influence on children's behavior may be mediated by parenting style. In a study of after-school behavior of latchkey children, children of authoritative parents had children who were less susceptible to engaging in risky behavior suggested by peers. This fits nicely with results provided by Pratt (1973), indicating that authoritative parents had children who engaged in the highest levels of preventive health behavior.

Adolescent High-Risk Behavior

Although a systematic review of the literature on adolescent high-risk behavior is beyond the scope of this book, it is important to present the major line of thought on the predictors and correlates of adolescent high-risk behavior, particularly in the context of peer influence on this type of behavior. A variety of theories have been developed and tested in an effort to account for the development of deviant behavior in adolescence, especially the use of alcohol and other drugs. There are two types of theories: those that consider the effects of alcohol and drug use and those concerned with the psychological and social factors associated with alcohol and drug use. Some theories of the first type stress the addictive qualities of these substances. It is generally accepted that these addiction theories are not adequate in explaining adolescent substance use, in part because relatively few adolescents consume enough alcohol and drugs to produce classical addiction (Bejerot, 1980; Oetting & Beauvais, 1987). Other theories of the first type are gateway theories focusing on the progressive use of substances (e.g., from tobacco use to marijuana use to hard drug use). These theories are also somewhat unsatisfactory in explaining adolescent substance use, because the perception that there is an orderly progression in substance use is probably attributable to such factors as availability and general attitudes toward their use (Oetting & Beauvais, 1987). Although these theories are helpful in suggesting that substance use is often associated with future substance use, a second group of theories, psychological and social theories, probably provide better explanations of adolescent substance use (Oetting & Beauvais, 1987). A huge number of studies have addressed the question of which social, cultural, and psychological factors place adolescents at risk for substance use. Social theories explain substance use as a function of underlying social problems and focus on minority youth (Lukoff, 1980). These theories have been criticized, however, for their limited generalizability to the vast population of adolescents across all ethnic and social groups who engage in substance use. Psychological theories stress the role of substances in satisfying the personality or life needs of adolescent users (Spotts & Schontz, 1984). Research using this model, however, has not been very successful in relating personality to substance use in adolescence. The third type of theory that has been developed to describe and predict adolescent substance use is psychosocial theory, which addresses both social environmental and person characteristics (Oetting & Beauvais, 1987). One of the most influential theories of this type has been the problem behavior theory of Jessor and his colleagues (Jessor, 1992).

A theory that particularly stresses the role of peers in adolescent deviance is peer cluster theory (Oetting & Beauvais, 1987). This theory, developed from surveys of over 15,000 minority and nonminority students, is based on the assumption that although other factors such as families and socioeconomic status may set the stage for alcohol and drug use, the initiation and maintenance of such use in adolescence is almost entirely a function of membership in peer clusters, small groups of people with whom the adolescent is identified. In other words, although other underlying social factors may render a child vulnerable, actual use of alcohol and other drugs almost always occurs through contact with peers. These authors suggest:

> When drugs are actually used, it is almost always in a peer context. Peers initiate the youth into drugs. Peers help provide drugs. Peers talk with each other about drugs and model drug-using behaviors for each other and in doing so shape attitudes about drugs and drug-using behaviors. A peer cluster consensus is reached about where and when drugs are to be used, about how much to use drugs, and even about how drugs affect you emotionally and how you behave when you take particular drugs. The influence of a peer cluster can also be positive – a group of friends can reject use of alcohol and drugs, and that group will together develop attitudes, values, and rationales that counter the use of drugs and alcohol. (p. 137)

Psychoimmunology of Peer Relationships

Stressful life events such as illness, the death of family members, family transitions such as divorce, or the birth of a sibling influence children's mental and physical health (Compas, Connor-Smith, Saltzman, & Thomsen, 2001; Rutter, 2000). It has long been argued that stress impacts immune system functioning, which in turn has consequences for individuals' physical health (Kiecolt-Glaser & Glaser, 1995).

At the same time, relationships can have a buffering effect on this stress–endocrine system–health linkage. Recent work by Kiecolt-Glaser and her colleagues, for example, suggests that marital satisfaction can protect couples from the adverse effects of stress (Kiecolt-Glaser & Glaser, 2001; Kiecolt-Glaser & Newton, 2001). A large body of research also demonstrates that social support from friends, neighbors, and coworkers can protect individuals from the adverse effects of stress (Sarason, Sarason, & Pierce, 1992). Peer relationships, especially close friendships, can serve a similar function for children. When a new infant joins a family, older siblings often exhibit a variety of stressful symptoms, such as regression, acting out, or jealousy. Kramer and Gottman (1992) found that 3- to 5-year-old children with close friendships experienced less stress than children without friends during the transition to sibship.

Berndt (1989) has provided some helpful guidelines for determining the conditions under which friendships function as buffers. First, friendships must survive the stressor in order to protect the individual. "Children with better friendships do not endure stressful events better than children with less adequate friendships if the stressful event separates children from their friends" (Parker, Rubin, Price, & DeRosier, 1995, p. 113). For example, children in families who relocate or who change schools may suffer loss of friendships, which is unfortunate because these transitions themselves are stressful events. Second, friendships are most effective when their support matches the child's needs. "When a child needs help with homework, a friend who answers questions about the assignment . . . may render more effective support than a friend who tries to make the child feel better about his or her abilities" (Berndt, 1989, p. 318). Third, just as in adult social support, it is important to distinguish between availability and utilization (Sarason et al., 1992) in children's friendships. The child must utilize the support of friends under stressful conditions (Asher, Rose, & Gabriel, 2001). Similarly, Sandler, Miller, Short, and Wolchik (1989) note the diverse ways in which friendships influence children's ability to cope with stress. First, friendship can prevent the occurrence of stressful events. Second, when stress is encountered, friends can play a moderating role by reducing the negative effects of the stressful experiences on the child. Finally, Sandler et al. note that friendship-based support enhances or improves the children's coping skills – which, in turn, buffer them against the negative impact of stressful events.

Are Parents and Peers Separate Influences?

Although we have treated family and peer influences as separate and independent, they often operate together in determining children's health outcomes. First, the relation between family and peer systems changes across development. In the preschool years, parents function as managers of children's social contact with peers (Ladd & LeSieur, 1995; Parke & Bhavnagri, 1989). For example, parental discussion about day care and preschool can later influence children's exposure to peers. As Ladd and LeSieur (1995, p. 390) note, "When parents enroll children in child care or preschool, they ensure access to a 'ready-made' peer group and a context in which children are typically encouraged to interact and make friends with peers." These opportunities to develop friendships – even in the preschool period – can have important effects on children's ability to cope with stressful change (e.g., Kramer & Gottman, 1992) and indirectly impact their health status.

Parents also influence children's health indirectly by their choice of neighborhood. Although microeconomic constraints often influence these choices, living in dangerous or crime-ridden neighborhoods can increase children's risk-related behaviors. Using census tract data, several investigators (Brooks-Gunn, Duncan, Klebanov, & Sealand, 1993; Coulton & Pandey, 1992) found that high-poverty areas were characterized by large numbers of low-birth-weight infants and high levels of juvenile delinquency.

It is commonly accepted that an authoritative childrearing style may be associated with positive social and health outcomes in children and youth living in low-risk neighborhoods (Baumrind, 1978; Steinberg, Lamborn, Dornbusch, & Darling, 1992). For example, Steinberg (1986), in a study of 865 adolescents, found that children of authoritative parents were less likely to succumb to peer influence. Some were at home after school or at a friend's house, whereas others described themselves as "hanging out," with little adult supervision. Children are more likely to be open to peer pressure when hanging out than at home. However, being reared authoritatively can protect children and make them less susceptible to peer influence, even when adult supervision is lax. Parenting style clearly generalizes to peer settings and can help children avoid being swayed by their peers to engage in health-threatening activities.

Recent research that takes into account the quality of the neighborhood has questioned the generalizability of the finding that authoritative parenting is always the best style. Families who reside in more dangerous and health-threatening neighborhoods may adapt their childrearing style to suit their current ecological conditions. In support of this view, Baldwin, Baldwin, and Cole (1990) found that poor minority parents who used more authoritarian childrearing practices had better-adjusted children than those relying on authoritative strategies. Although these strategies may minimize children's risk-taking behaviors by keeping them out of contact with deviant peers, as Steinberg's (1986) work suggests, when parental surveillance is minimal, peer influence may increase in families that use authoritarian childrearing. These findings underscore the need to develop models that recognize the roles of multiple socialization agents in promoting children's health (Tinsley et al., 2002).

Summing Up

Thus, it appears that although family influence is still important during adolescence with respect to health behavior, peer influence is significant as well, although the interaction is complex and not yet clearly understood. More work is necessary to clarify under what conditions and with what types of health behaviors peers or parents are relatively influential.

In health behavior, the influence of peers, especially in young children and with respect to normative health behavior, is unexamined. In light of the significant influence of peers in other developmental domains, as discussed earlier, it is clear that peer processes must affect young children's health behavior, at least during the preschool and early elementary years. Exploration of peer processes, situational and individual difference modifying factors, and their effects on children's health behavior would appear to be a critical extension of our models of the development of children's health behavior.

Schools as Influences on Children's Health

Schools have a significant influence on children's health behavior (American Academy of Pediatrics, 2000b). Effective school-based health education teaches children what healthful and unhealthful behaviors are and the consequences of these behaviors (Lightfoot & Bines, 2000; Sarafino, 1990). Moreover, schools are the usual setting for extrafamilial interventions designed to modify children's health attitudes and behaviors. Schools are attractive for these purposes for a number of reasons, including their inclusivity (almost all U.S. children attend school in the early grades) and the young ages at which children begin school. The young age of school children is important; their health habits must be affected early, before maladaptive health behavior becomes ingrained (Taylor, 1999). School-based health education can help children avoid developing unhealthful habits when they are most vulnerable, and help them acquire health-protective behaviors that become a habitual aspect of their beliefs and lifestyles (Sarafino, 1990).

School-Based Health Education Programs

In the preschool and early elementary years, surprisingly few efforts have been made to teach children preventive health attitudes and behavior. This may be due to the assumption that children are not cognitively ready for this type of instruction, especially as proposed by those endorsing the stage theory of children's acquisition of health-related knowledge. For the most part, early childhood educators are not prepared to teach children about health. Few preschools or elementary schools have health educators or a health curriculum, and when these do exist, they are focused on specific health issues such as substance use or, more recently, AIDS (Midford & McBride, 2001; Sussman, 2001). One of the messages children receive from these programs is that an appropriate (e.g., teacher-sanctioned) approach to health is problem- and crisis-related. Children do not learn in their early school years that preventive health facts and skill development are important (Mellanby, Rees, & Tripp, 2000).

There are, however, health programs designed for preschools, and several quality preschool curricula have been developed and evaluated (Parcel, Bruhn, & Murray, 1983). One such program is "Hale and Hardy's Helpful Health Hints," a preschool health education program. Pre- and posttesting of children's health knowledge indicated that children exposed to the program, which focused on the five senses, safety, nutrition, dental health, personal responsibility, emotions, hygiene, and drugs/medicine, increased their health knowledge significantly more than a control group of children. This study provides further evidence of the modifiability of health knowledge. Unfortunately, concomitant changes in the preschoolers' health behavior were not measured in this study.

One health domain, cardiovascular health, has been the focus of several studies on school health education programs for older children. A review of school-based cardiovascular research suggests that school-based programs are effective in changing children's knowledge of nutrition and their intention to smoke cigarettes, but changes in behavior are more difficult to achieve. Several studies illustrate the potential value of these programs, as well as the range of change agents that can be utilized in schools. Typically, in these studies, prevention and intervention focus on one health behavior, such as nutrition (Ellison, Capper, Goldberg, Witschi, & Stare, 1989; Luepker, Perry, Murray, & Mullis, 1988) and blood pressure reduction (Fors, Owen, Hall, McLaughlin, & Levinson, 1980). Ellison and colleagues, using the food service staff, focused on lowering the fat and sodium content of food served at two private boarding schools. Using recipe analysis and biochemical analysis of food items, they demonstrated that the fat and sodium content of the food could be lowered. In this study, teachers were utilized to help sixth-grade children lower their blood pressure. In addition, the students were required to teach their parents about high blood pressure. Changes in knowledge and in monitoring blood pressure were found as a result of the intervention.

Parcel and his colleagues (Parcel, Simons-Morton, O'Hara, Baranowski, & Wilson, 1989) and Nader and his colleagues (Perry, Sellers, Johnson, & Pedersen, 1997) examined induced changes in children's nutrition and physical activity. Both programs reported positive changes in knowledge as well as shifts in diet (e.g., total fat, saturated fat, complex carbohydrate intake); the Nader et al. program found changes in cholesterol and blood pressure as well.

Other studies were designed to modify children's smoking or weight control, in addition to their nutrition and physical activity (Killen et al., 1989; Marcoux, Sallis, McKenzie, & Marshall, 1999; Perry et al., 1997; Walter, 1989; Weinberg, Carbonari, & Laufman, 1984). In these school-based programs, curriculum components were often combined with environmental change and family home-based participation. The most successful of these programs appear to emphasize skill change as well as knowledge change, focus on many aspects of children's environment (i.e., cafeteria, home, and snacks in nutrition-focused programs), use intervention provider training, and use multiple measures of outcome or change (see Stone, Perry, & Luepker, 1989, for a detailed review of these studies).

Although earlier critics such as Bartlett (1981) offered pessimistic assessments of the impact of school-based health education on children's health attitudes and behavior, these more recent programs suggest that health-related change can be achieved. These programs remain most effective in modifying health knowledge, but progress has been made in changing health attitudes and behavior as well (O'Donnell, Stueve, Doval, & Duran, 1999). Stone and colleagues (Stone et al., 1989) have offered a variety of suggestions for improving curriculum-based health interventions. These include the following: "emphasis on the utility of theory-based health curriculum and intervention development including the identification of psychosocial risk factors...and recognition of the need to continue both small efficacy studies as well as effectiveness and diffusion research studies in the school health field" (p. 166).

Bartlett (1981), in a critical evaluation of the published outcome studies of traditional school health education programs concerning drugs and alcohol, smoking, nutrition, driver education, dental health, and heart health, suggests that school-based health education could be significantly improved. Although these programs are fairly effective in modifying health knowledge, they are less effective in changing health attitudes and mostly ineffective in modifying health behavior. Bartlett cites philosophical differences in communities regarding the appropriateness of various health topics for inclusion in school-based health programs and the group format of these programs as possible reasons for their general ineffectiveness in changing health behavior.

Schools as Health-Care Delivery Sites

Schools are being used not only to present health intervention and prevention programs but also, as Joy Dryfoos argues in her 1994 book *Full Service Schools*, to deliver health and other services to children and youth. There are three types of health services provisions in schools: school-based, school-linked, and community-based (Carlson, Tharinger, Bricklin, & DeMers, 1996; Dryfoos, 1994; Fothergill & Ballard, 1998; Hacker & Wessel, 1998; Klostermann, Perry, & Britto, 2000). School-based approaches consist of comprehensive health service systems. School-linked models have been described as "those provided through a collaboration among schools, health care providers and social service agencies" (DeMers & Bricklin, 1995, p. 219). Finally, community-based services are generally located outside the school and managed by nonschool personnel (e.g., departments of mental health or parks and recreation facilities) (Fothergill & Ballard, 1998).

Several recent models of health service delivery illustrate both the recent shifts in this area and the potential impact of schools as sites for influencing children's health attitudes and behavior. DeMers & Bricklin (1995) describe several models of school-based health care. One influential model developed by the Robert Wood Johnson Foundation is the school-based health clinic. Although these clinics began in high schools to target the health risk behaviors of adolescents, they have recently expanded in number, scope, and school level. In the 1980s, school-based health care expanded rapidly and by 1991 was found in nearly every state. According to Dryfoos (1994), these clinics number nearly 600. Their scope has broadened to include school dropout, substance abuse, and mental health problems as well as prevention, health promotion, and treatment. And no longer are they restricted to high schools; they are increasingly evident in elementary and middle schools (DeMers & Bricklin, 1995).

Although evaluation data indicate that these programs are being utilized by the targeted students, and increase access to health care for these students (Dowden, Calvert, Davis, & Gullotta, 1997), the impact of these clinics on children's health outcomes is less clear (Weist, 2001).

Another example is the model utilized in Kentucky, which represents a statewide effort to link education and health care reform. Through the Kentucky Education Reform Act (KERA) of 1990, health and social centers were established on nearly all elementary and high school sites in which 20% of the students were eligible for free lunch. The goal was to provide programs for children and youth at risk for school failure due to economic disadvantage, limited health and social services, substance abuse, and family stress. Services range from referrals to health and social services and substance abuse counseling to family-oriented services such as parent training, social support, and ensuring access to community resources. Evaluation of the program suggests that nearly 19,000 families have been served (Kalafat & Illback, 1998), with teachers and school administrators accounting for nearly 50% of the referrals. Health problems accounted for over 21% of the referrals; behavior, emotional, and school-related problems (e.g., dropout risk, poor attendance, discipline problems) accounted for the remainder. Families report high satisfaction with the Kentucky Clinic program; dramatic decreases in psychiatric hospitalizations and increases in social support to families are other results attributed to the program (Kalafat & Illback, 1998). The direct impact on children's health is less clear, but as our model outlined in Chapter 8 argues, improved family functioning is likely to be associated with decreased health risk.

Summing Up

There has been a significant expansion of the use of schools for the delivery of health-related services for children and adolescents over the past decade. The early evaluations of these programs are positive, but it is too early to conclude that they will significantly influence children's health status. Even less clear is whether they alter children's health attitudes and behaviors. The next step is to integrate classroom-based health promotion programs with these health service delivery efforts. Both components are necessary to prevent the development of poor health habits and to increase utilization of health services if early preventive efforts are not fully successful. School-based health education remains a potentially strong factor in the socialization of children's health behavior. Further research is required to determine how these programs can be more effective in helping children acquire wellness-promoting behavior.

7

How Television Viewing and Other Media Use Affect Children's Health

Parents, schools, and peers are not the only influences on children's health; television viewing and other media use helps shape children's health attitudes and behavior (Anderson, Huston, Schmitt, Linebarger, & Wright, 2001). In an era when researchers, policymakers, and media industrialists are attempting to sort out the complex relations between children and mass media, the entire nature of media is undergoing dramatic change. The explosive growth of the Internet and computer technology, as well as access to these, is ushering in a new media culture that is being embraced wholeheartedly by children and adolescents (Montgomery, 2000). A recent survey of youths' use of all types of media (television, videotapes, movies, computers, video games, radio, compact discs, tape players, books, newspapers, magazines) suggests that children and adolescents are immersed in these media forms (Roberts, 2000). Most households contain most types of media, and the majority of youth own their own. The average American child devotes almost 7 hours per day to media use (Roberts, 2000). Television is the dominant form, although about one-half of children and adolescents use computers daily.

During an average year, an American child will watch a variety of events on television that have clear implications for health and health risk: almost 2,000 commercials for alcohol, more than 14,000 sexual references, and more than 1,000 murders, rapes, and assaults (Strasburger, 1989; Strasburger & Donnerstein, 2000; Strasburger & Hendrin, 1995). Children and adolescents spend more time watching television than any other activity except sleeping, and more time from ages 2 to 18 watching television (15,000–18,000 hours) than they spend in classrooms (12,000 hours) (Byrd-Bredbenner & Grasso, 2000; Levin, 1998; Montgomery,

2000; Roberts, 2000; Strasburger, 1992; Strasburger & Hendrin, 1995). On average, youth aged 12–17 years watch television for 3–5 hours, and children aged 2–11 years watch television for nearly $3\frac{1}{2}$ hours per day (Strasburger & Donnerstein, 2000). By the time today's children reach age 70, they will have spent about 7 years of their lives watching television.

The impact of television on children's attitudes and behavior has been well documented over the past 30 years. Consistent viewing of aggressive and risk-taking behavior – often without clear negative consequences – has been linked to aggressive and antisocial behavior, as well as other health-threatening behaviors, in both children and adults (Bryant & Bryant, 2001; Frydman, 1999; Huesmann, Eron, Lefkowitz, & Walder, 1984; Huston & Wright, 1998; Singer & Singer, 2000; Winston, Duyck Wolff, Jordan, & Bhatia, 2000). Additionally, given the pervasiveness of soap operas and other sexually provocative and explicit television programming, it is not surprising that children's sexual attitudes and behavior are also modified by television viewing. Finally, programs portraying risk-taking and suicide impacts on youths' attitudes and behavior as well.

The content of television programs is not the only culprit to be identified in the relations between television viewing and health-risky behavior; commercials are a powerful influence on children's health (Byrd-Bredbenner & Grasso, 2000; DeJong & Hoffman, 2000; Unnikrishnan & Bajpai, 1996; Winston, Duyck Wolff, Jordan, & Bhatia, 2000); experts estimate that American children view approximately 20,000 television commercials each year (Strasburger, 1989, 1995). Billions of dollars are spent each year by corporations to televise commercial advertisements for non-nutritional foods such as sugary cereals, candy, and high-fat fast foods that are attractive to children. Of all the broadcasting media, American television is the most commercially exploitive of children in the Western world (Charren, 1985). It is not only food commercials that affect children's health; advertisements for medicine influence their health attitudes and behavior as well.

Not only does television directly influence children's health through its programs and commercials; television has an indirect effect as well by changing children's lifestyles. Their recreational choices, activity levels, and other determinants of health have been linked to television watching (Frydman, 1999). Before we turn to a more detailed discussion of these issues, let's examine the ways in which children learn from television.

How Children Learn from Television

One of the most important ways in which children learn is through modeling the attitudes and behaviors of adults and older children (Anderson et al., 2001; Bandura, 1989; Huston & Wright, 1996). Television provides a plethora of such models. As Strasburger (1992) observes:

> Although instances of direct imitation are relatively rare, television acts more insidiously to shape viewers' attitudes and perceptions of social norms. For older children and adolescents, television can give direct access to the formerly secret adult world to which they were rarely privy. Older children and adolescents can learn new "scripts" about gender roles, conflict resolution, and patterns of adult courtship and sexual gratification. (p. 144)

The potency of television viewing for modifying behavior and attitudes has been well documented in classic studies of the detrimental impact of television violence on children's aggression, as well as the beneficial effects of prosocial and educational programming (Huston et al., 1992) and even more recent literature (Bryant & Bryant, 2001; Singer & Singer, 2000). Even more relevant for understanding television's impact on children's health are a series of studies by Potts and his colleagues (Potts, Doppler, & Hernandez, 1994; Potts, Runyan, Zerger, & Marchetti, 1996; Potts & Swisher, 1998), which document that watching television programs depicting risk-taking behavior increases children's self-reported physical risk-taking in hypothetical situations. Specifically, after viewing selected edited commercial television programs shown on Saturday mornings depicting high risk-taking, children aged 6–9 reported they would take more risk in such situations as climbing trees, retrieving a ball from the street, approaching a flaming barbecue grill, and so on than they had reported in a pretest of similar but unique risk situations.

Although safety behaviors are modeled on television programs that are popular with child audiences, most are performed by male characters, have limited salience for children, and are not associated with either positive or negative repercussions. As Potts and his colleagues (1996) concluded:

> [B]ased on social learning principles pertaining to observational learning, the models in this sample of programs [depicting safety behaviors] do not demonstrate consistently successful behaviors or behaviors with relevance to child viewers.... Because most [of the safety behaviors] were performed as precautions, rather than in

response to immediate danger, few of those behaviors were followed by either positive or negative consequences. Thus the utility of the modeled safety behaviors may not be apparent to young viewers. (p. 524)

Not only does television provide fascinating models for children, but children take the behaviors of these models very seriously. Why? The Institute for Mental Health Initiatives (1996) suggests four reasons. First, children are perpetually searching for new models of behavior beyond their families. Television characters, in conjunction with other outside socialization agents (e.g., teachers, coaches, other adults), become powerful models of attitudes and behavior. Second, because children want to be socially accepted by their peers, they are highly receptive to televised messages about how to fit in and be accepted by others. Televised programs are an important contribution to the definition of contemporary peer culture. Third, as children develop cognitively, they are increasingly aware of the ideas and attitudes of others, including those expressed by television characters (Carlson, Laczniak, & Walsh, 2001). Finally, developing children are expanding their social skills, perceptions of their responsibilities, and behavioral repertoires of limit-setting (Greene, Rubin, Hale, & Walters, 1996). Television often provides quick and easy answers to the difficult work of establishing and maintaining relationships with others. However, the impact of these answers may depend on the developmental status of the child viewer. Research- and theory-based information about how children think or reason about health-related behavior and risk demonstrates how the content and delivery of these health messages affect children's responses to televised material (Greene et al., 1996).

Research over the past 20 years has shown that young children have difficulty separating televised fact from fiction. This suggests that the knowledge that most televised entertainment programming is fiction develops slowly over the elementary school years. However, even by the end of elementary school, about one-third of boys still do not completely understand that television characters are fictional and played by actors (Gunter & McAleer, 1990).

In fact, even adults' views of reality are shaped by television. George Gerbner, a renowned communications expert (Gerbner, Gross, Morgan, & Signorielli, 1980), has proposed that the more a person is exposed to television, the more likely the person's perceptions of reality will match those depicted on television. This *cultivation* theory suggests that people who spend more time watching television are more likely to perceive the real world in ways that reflect the messages delivered on television than people who watch less television (Comstock & Paik, 1991). Morgan (1988) suggests that many aspects of people's attitudes and beliefs are altered by television in this manner, including ideas about aggression and violence, sex roles, occupations, science, education, minorities, family life, politics, and, of course, children's and adults' health. Thus, in addition to offering children and adolescents attractive and exciting role models, television profoundly influences children by providing a frame through which they can interpret their experiences. George Comstock, a leading researcher on the effects of television on both children and adults, suggests that although real life is the primary source of most experience, television is very salient, particularly to children and adolescents, because it provides nonredundant information. Comstock and Paik (1991) state: "Television programming is filled with images and experiences not available locally to most young viewers. When programs pertain to knowledge, beliefs, and perceptions for which alternative sources have been absent, television may function as a source of information" (pp. 186–187).

For example, research findings suggest that boys who were heavy television viewers were somewhat more likely than those who watched less television to overestimate the amount of violence in their neighborhoods and in the world, even if they had never experienced violence themselves (Gerbner, Gross, Signorielli, Morgan, & Jackson-Beeck, 1979). Moreover, the children who had experienced violence themselves and those who had merely watched a lot of violence on television had more or less the same worldview about the existence of violence in society.

For some, television viewing becomes a substitute for reality. In light of earlier work on aggression (Coie & Dodge, 1998; Dodge, 1985), it is possible to conclude that frequent television viewers would develop the expectation that other people have hostile intentions – a view that is linked to heightened aggression and, of course, an increased risk of harm and injury.

Are children's views of physical health affected in similar ways? According to Lewis and Lewis's (1974) study of the effects of television on health behavior of fifth- and sixth-grade children, the answer is clearly yes. These researchers studied the effects of television commercials on the children's health behavior. Forty-seven percent of the children accepted all the health-related messages in the commercials as completely truthful and 70% believed the messages, at least in part (Lewis & Lewis, 1974; Liebert & Sprafkin, 1988). This finding is particularly chilling in light of the authors' report that a panel of experts found 70% of the messages to be inaccurate, misleading, or both. Clearly, not only do children learn specific health lessons and behaviors from television, but their inability to distinguish fantasy from reality in televised portrayals may produce misleading and potentially health-threatening views of the real world.

The Effects of Television Viewing on Children's Nutrition

One of the major health hazards for children is their high consumption of low-nutrition foods, which is linked with obesity, dental problems, and lower consumption of more nutritious foods (Armstrong et al., 1998). Long-term exposure to commercials for low-nutrition foods (i.e., foods high in sugar, such as soda, and/or high in fat, such as french fries) has a significant influence on children's eating behavior (Liebert & Sprafkin, 1988; Unnikrishnan & Bajpai, 1996; Wilson, Quigley, & Mansoor, 1999). Commercials for low-nutrition foods comprise approximately 80% of children's televised advertising (Barcus, 1987). Information about food and eating on television is not restricted to commercials; in fact, studies indicate that there are more food-related references in programs than in commercials (Kaufman, 1980). Eating, drinking, or talking about food occurs more than nine times per hour in prime-time and weekend daytime programming (Gerbner, Gross, Morgan, & Signorielli, 1981). Snacking represents 39% of the portrayals of eating during these time periods, and representations of healthful snacking are virtually absent. Few television characters ever eat carrot sticks or munch on apples.

Several studies have examined the links between children's eating behavior, body images, and media images of beauty (Anderson et al., 2001; Jambor, 2001). A study of the relations between the use of electronic media and the perceived importance of appearance and weight concerns among adolescent girls examined television, videotape, video and computer game, and music video use (Borzekowski, Robinson, & Killen, 2000). While total use of these media was not related to the girls' perceived importance of appearance and weight, girls who watched more music videos believed their appearance to be more important and had more weight concerns than girls who watched fewer music videos. These results suggest that frequent music video viewing may cause girls to be overly concerned about their appearance and weight, both of which have been linked to girls' disordered eating.

Among early elementary school children, television viewing predicted an increased trend in boys' stereotyping of female characters as fat

(Harrison, 2000a). Similar patterns were also demonstrated in older children, with exposure to fat characters on television predicting girls' eating disorder symptoms (Harrison, 2000a). For both boys and girls, television viewing predicted greater eating disorder symptoms (Harrison, 2000a). As children's television viewing hours increased each week, so did their number of eating disorder symptoms.

How television influences children's disordered eating is not completely understood. However, dieting to lose weight is a norm, in society in general and on television specifically. Children may not innately or naturally favor thin body types, but they may engage in television-influenced dieting and exercise prior to internalizing the message that a thin body is a socially ideal body (Jambor, 2001) and may later regard dieting as a glamorous, "grown-up" behavior to be emulated.

Studies indicate that television characters are usually happy in the presence of food, yet food is usually not used to satisfy hunger in television programs. Instead, it is used to bribe others or to facilitate social interactions (Kaufman, 1980). The uncoupling of food from hunger could undermine children's learning of the links between internal cues and eating behavior – a deficit that scientists have argued is one of the conditions leading to obesity and other eating disorders (Friedman & Brownell, 1995).

Studies suggest that these ads substantially affect the attitudes and behaviors of children with respect to nutrition and food selection (Byrd-Bredbenner & Grasso, 2000; Hammond, Wyllie, & Casswell, 1999). Of 269 commercials for food embedded in a sample of programming, 73% were for foods high in fat or sugar (Wilson et al., 1999). The authors of this study suggest that children who ate only those foods would have a diet too high in fat, saturated fat, protein, sugar, and sodium and too low in fiber and a variety of minerals and vitamins, including vitamin E, magnesium, and selenium. The authors concluded that televised food commercials increase the risks of obesity in childhood, and of dental problems, diabetes, cardiovascular disease, and cancer in adulthood.

Studies have determined that young children (4 to 7 years old) do not understand that sugary foods are detrimental to health, nor are the cautions presented in these commercials effective (e.g., ads for sugary cereals stating that they should be part of a balanced breakfast) (Liebert & Sprafkin, 1988; Strasburger, 1995). Just as children are unable to comprehend the links between violent or criminal behavior and its consequences on television, they are also unable to comprehend the often low-key and less salient disclaimer messages that are often "tacked on" to strident and powerful ads for Sugar Pops, Froot Loops, and Lucky Charms. Although television consistently presents characters who are thin (with 88% of all television characters thin or average in weight), it is ironic that the nutritional products and behaviors most heavily advertised on television promote obesity (Kaufman, 1980; Strasburger, 1992, 1995).

Nor are the advertisers wasting their money. Children's food selections are influenced by television commercials – further testimony to the impact of television on children's health-related behavior. Studies of children's actual food selection, as influenced by television commercials, underscore the potency of television's impact on this child health behavior. Experimental studies of exposure to commercials of low-nutrition foods reveal that children choose more low-nutrition and fewer high-nutrition foods (Gorn & Greenberg, 1982), especially boys (Jeffrey, McClerran, & Fox, 1982). Field studies of the relation between children's television viewing and nutritional status yield similar findings: a linear relation between television viewing and poor nutritional habits and nutrition misconceptions. Children who are heavy viewers are more likely to believe that a healthy breakfast consists of sugared cereals and that fast food is nutritious (Signorielli & Lears, 1992). In light of many studies demonstrating that there are serious consequences to children of even mild protein-energy malnutrition and a mildly poor diet, these connections between television viewing and diet are alarming. For example, children on protein-deficient diets have less energy, poorer social skills, and impaired academic achievement (Sigman, 1995).

Television commercials about food also affect the self-perception of children who are overweight (Anderson et al., 2001). Nine- and 10-year-old British children's ratings of their own health was lower after they watched television advertisements for sweet snacks if the children were overweight. This suggests that more attention should be devoted to identifying how the characteristics of the children and the features of the advertising influence the effectiveness of the ads.

Television can have positive effects, and its resources potentially can be utilized to improve children's nutritional habits (Huston et al., 1992). However, pronutritional advertising is less successful in modifying behavior than in changing cognitive understanding; nutrition knowledge increases, but consumption patterns do not change (Peterson, Jeffrey, Bridgewater, & Dawson, 1984). Pronutritional programming can be successful when combined with positive evaluative comments by an adult coviewer, such as the child's father; it can be effective in reducing 3- to

6-year-old children's consumption of low-nutrition foods (Galst, 1980; St. Peters, Fitch, Huston, & Wright, 1991). Together, these studies suggest at least the powerful potential of children's viewing of nutrition-related television advertising.

"I'd Rather Watch TV": The Indirect Impact of Children's Television Viewing on Their Activity Choices

Children's television viewing has an effect on children's health behavior beyond program influence: It alters time use and activity choices in children (Armstrong et al., 1998; Robinson, 1972; Strasburger, 1992). A recent survey by *Prevention* magazine (Princeton Survey Research Associates, 1994) found that whereas children spend approximately 18 hours a week watching television (equal to 2 months of waking hours per year), parents report that 66% of children get only 20 minutes of strenuous exercise at least three times per week. Williams and Handford (1986) found that the number of sports activities (i.e., health-promoting exercise) engaged in by adolescents markedly decreased after the introduction of television into the community. The consequences of these shifts are illustrated in a study by Hei and Gold (1990), which found that children who watch television for 2 to 4 hours a day had dramatically higher cholesterol levels than those who watched it for less than 2 hours per day. This effect is probably mediated by insufficient exercise and television-related snacking on high-fat foods. Other studies confirm these findings, demonstrating that children who watch the most television have more body fat and higher body mass indices than those who watch much less television (Andersen, Crespo, Bartlett, Cheskin, & Pratt, 1998). Kubey and Csikszentmihalyi (1990) found that one-quarter to one-third of the time that families watch television, they eat as well. The number of hours spent watching television is a strong predictor of childhood and adolescent obesity, with the prevalence increasing 2% for each hour viewed above the norm (Dietz & Gortmaker, 1985). And, as scientists have documented, unfit, obese children appear to be at increased risk, in comparison to their more fit counterparts, for high cholesterol, due primarily to high body fat, resulting in adult atherosclerosis and other life-threatening cardiovascular diseases (Armstrong et al., 1998).

Many studies have documented the relations among children's television viewing, children's activity levels, and childhood obesity over the last few years. Television viewing appears to be inextricably linked, in a positive linear fashion, with less physical activity, greater consumption of high-fat and sugared foods, lower consumption of healthy foods, and obesity (Armstrong et al., 1998; Crooks, 2000; Epstein, Paluch, Gordy, & Dorn, 2000; Hanley et al., 2000; Hernandez et al., 1999; Lindquist et al., 1999; Tanasecu, Ferris, Himmelgreen, Rodriguez, & Perez-Escamilla, 2000; Woodring, 1998). These studies have examined these links throughout the United States and in many other countries, including Puerto Rico, Canada, Australia, New Zealand, Mexico, Great Britain, and Italy.

As these studies suggest, these effects appear to derive from their substitution of television viewing for more health-promoting types of recreational activity, the portrayal of poor nutritional behavior, the advertisement of low-nutrition products, or some combination of all of these factors (Strasburger, 1992; Strasburger & Donnerstein, 2000). The direction-of-effects issue is still open. Although it is implied that television viewing may lead to eating patterns that are directly linked to obesity, it is also plausible that obese children may be less likely to play actively and therefore watch more television (Lindquist et al., 1999). In light of recent evidence suggesting that childhood obesity is strongly related to negative self-concept and depression, these relations between children's television viewing, physical activity, and child outcomes are particularly troubling (Kolody & Sallis, 1995).

The Effects of Children's Television Viewing on Medicine and Drug Use

Other health-related effects of children's television viewing concern programs depicting substance use and commercials for medicine (Anderson et al., 2001). Although very little medical television advertising is aimed specifically at children, children view these commercials frequently (Almarsdottir & Zimmer, 1998; Liebert & Sprafkin, 1988). Research on such viewing by children has focused on legal and illicit substance use. Children's viewing of ads for medicine have been linked with their requests for and use of these drugs, although the effects are weak to moderate (Liebert & Sprafkin, 1988; Rossiter & Robertson, 1980). However, in light of the high rates of unsupervised self-medication by young children (Iannotti & Bush, 1992) involving both over-the-counter and prescription medicines, even modest links between television viewing of medicine commercials and use of these medicines is important.

Television depicts risky behaviors such as substance use as socially acceptable, with an important impact on children's health behavior. Further, these depictions of risky behavior and its consequences on television imply that the health consequences of these behaviors are a matter of "beating the odds." Although available research does not suggest that children's use of illicit drugs is affected by viewing commercials for legal drugs (Milovsky, Pekowsky, & Stipp, 1975–1976), other related concerns remain. In light of young children's perceived invulnerability to negative health outcomes (Gochman, 1987), the media's tendency to publicize individuals who "beat the odds" can be construed as further encouragement for children to take risks (Bruhn & Cordova, 1977; Potts et al., 1996; Winston et al., 2000).

Over the past 40 years, researchers have attempted to pinpoint the influence of media on child and adolescent alcohol use (Anderson et al., 2001). These studies repeatedly suggest that these influences are complex, interactive, and difficult to separate from other sources of influence such as the alcohol use in children's homes (Resnick, 1990). However, we do know that children and adolescents are frequently exposed to alcohol advertising. Strasburger (1990, 1992, 1995) reported that beer and wine producers spend more than $900 million each year on advertising, including television commercials. This type of advertising outnumbers substance use counteradvertising by 25:1 to 50:1 (Atkin, 1990) and delivers the message that alcohol use is "fun, sexy, likely to make you sexier or more popular, and has no bad repercussions" (Strasburger, 1992, p. 148). Other work identifies children's repetitive exposure to television characters engaged in sipping alcohol, displaying drunken behavior, and making jokes about drinking, particularly in sitcoms, as a *latent function*, which describes how messages about alcohol and drinking are sent to viewers by television programmers without either realizing or intending to participate in a process of alcohol education (de Foe & Breed, 1988).

Research demonstrates that televised alcohol ads are effective with youth. For example, in a large sample of fifth and sixth graders in the United States, Grube and Wallack (1994) evaluated children's awareness of beer advertising on television. They asked the children to (1) identify brands of beer from photographs of currently televised beer advertisements without brand identification, (2) name as many brands of beer as possible without prompting, and (3) match beer slogans with their correct brands. Awareness was related to more knowledge of beer brands and slogans, more positive beliefs about beer drinking, and increased intentions to drink beer later in life (Grube & Wallack, 1994). In Sweden, which has banned such advertising for over 30 years, per capita consumption of alcohol has decreased 20%, while in the United States it has increased 50%

since 1960 (Romelsjo, 1987; Strasburger, 1990, 1995). Although it is clear that television is not the only factor that may contribute to children's consumption of alcohol and other drugs, these studies suggest that television advertising and programming may be playing a role in altering drinking patterns. Another issue that has been investigated is this: What does the individual child or adolescent bring to television viewing that affects how this viewing impacts him or her? Borzekowski (1996) examined the effects of two sitcoms popular with youthful viewers and still available regularly on cable television channels (*Family Matters* and *The Cosby Show*) with storylines depicting adolescents who drink too much alcohol and suffer the consequences of a bad hangover. The findings from this study suggest that knowing others who drink alcohol, regardless of whether they are friends, family, or acquaintances, does not significantly influence how students view negative alcohol messages. However, personal experience with drinking alcohol does impact the students' perception of these messages. Adolescents in this study who had little or no experience with alcohol reported more interest in these sitcom episodes than students with more experience with alcohol. How can this be explained? Perhaps adolescents who drink less find this programming more interesting because they are less familiar with situations involving alcohol. Alternatively, students who do drink may be disenchanted with antialcohol programs because they present evidence contrary to their own beliefs about using alcohol during adolescence (Borzekowski, 1996). Thus, this research suggests that students who regularly use alcohol during adolescence pay less attention to antialcohol messages on television. It might be argued that antialcohol programming is at least as important, if not more important, for teens who are not drinking alcohol or for those who are only at the experimental stage. However, more attention to ways of reaching those who are already drinking is needed if efforts to decrease alcohol use in adolescence are to be effective.

Television and Sexuality

By preadolescence, children are beginning to explore their own sexuality, and are interested in how their bodies work and in sexual behavior (Institute for Mental Health Initiatives, 1996). Children learn more about sexual behavior from the media than from their parents (Institute for Mental Health Initiatives, 1996; Zillman & Vorderer, 2000). The new media technology gives children and adolescents ready access to all types of erotica (Zillman & Vorderer, 2000).

Sexual content is a television staple (Brown & Hayes, 2001). It appears in more than half (56%) of all programs, and an average of 3.2 scenes per hour in television shows contain sexual content (Kunkel et al., 1999). In an average year, an American child is exposed to more than 14,000 sexual references, innuendoes, and jokes compared to fewer than 175 cautionary references to birth control, sexual self-control, abstinence, or STDs (Strasburger & Donnerstein, 1999).

The importance of television as a source of information for children and adolescents about sex is underscored by the inadequate teachings of parents and schools. Recent reports document that only one-fourth to one-half of parents talk comprehensively to their children about sex, and only one-third of schools provide detailed sex education (Huston & Wright, 1996; Strasburger, 1989, 1992, 1995). Fifty-three percent of the girls interviewed in one study reported getting their sex education from television. However, few studies have conclusively linked children's viewing of sexually oriented television programming to sexual behavior. A report by Princeton Survey Research Associates for the Henry J. Kaiser Family Foundation (1994) suggests that a third of adolescents believe that some youth have sex because television makes it seem normal.

The Alan Guttmacher Institute analyzed adolescent pregnancy rates worldwide. It found that although American adolescents are not more sexually active than their counterparts in Canada and Europe, the United States has the highest rate of adolescent pregnancy among the industrialized nations (Blum, 2001). The report attributed this finding, in part, to the way in which U.S. television portrays sexuality.

What are children and adolescents learning about sexuality from television? Although much more research is needed, we know a little about the effects of sex-related programming on youth (Ward & Rivadeneyra, 1999). Studies demonstrate that television appears to have a dramatic effect on children's and adolescents' beliefs about sexuality. For example, sexually active adolescents who think television characters are more proficient and enjoy sex more than they do are less satisfied with their own sexual experiences (Brown, Childers, & Waszak, 1990). Adolescents who watch many television programs depicting sexuality are more likely to have had sexual intercourse in the preceding year, although we cannot be sure whether sexual behavior causes the interest in sexual programming or vice versa (Brown & Newcomer, 1991).

Two aspects of sex-oriented programming affect children and adolescents: the inappropriate depiction of sexuality and the failure to portray responsible sexuality. With regard to the inappropriate portrayal of sexuality, Strasburger (1992) notes that on television "sex is used to sell everything from cars to shampoo, and when human sexuality is displayed irresponsibly, children and adolescents derive important cues about adult behavior" (p. 147). Television networks have been very reticent to allow birth control commercials, and when they are permitted, they focus on their efficacy in preventing pregnancy rather than STDs including AIDS.

Zillman (2000) reminds us of another media source of sexual information for children: the Internet:

> In the absence of acceptable forms of sex education in the schools, the conventional media, now supplemented by the Internet, are *de facto* providing sex education for our children and adolescents. The Internet, in particular, ensures ready access to all conceivable forms of sexual material, and any effective curtailment of such liberal access is unlikely. Children who are naturally curious about sexual matters are confronted with a barrage of information in which educational messages are bound to be overwhelmed by sexual adult entertainment from the common to the bizarre and aberrant. In view of this situation, few observers would argue that preschool children and first to fourth graders would have the cognitive and emotional maturity to separate the wheat from the chaff. (p. 42)

Television programs influence another aspect of children's sexuality, namely, the stereotypes they develop for physical beauty, particularly for girls (Harrison, 2000a, 2000b; Jambor, 2001). Preadolescent and adolescent girls in the United States spend an estimated $4 billion per year on cosmetics (Graham & Hamdan, 1987). By the end of high school, more than half of them have been on a "serious" diet, and a significant number of girls as young as 14 years of age have had breast reduction or enlargement surgery (Brown et al., 1990; Freedman, 1984). Content analyses of television programming suggest that the current standard of attractiveness portrayed by television is the slimmest for both women and men since the last epidemic of eating disorders in the 1920s (Silverstein, Peterson, & Perdue, 1986). The extreme ideals of physical and sexual attractiveness portrayed on television may exacerbate the difficulty many adolescents have in accepting their bodies and finding them attractive. Children whose bodies do not match the cultural ideal promoted by television, and by Western society more generally, are at increased risk for depression, low self-esteem, excessive use of cosmetics, excessive cosmetic surgery, preoccupation with weight loss, eating disorders, and engaging in sexual activity for the purpose of self-validation (Brown et al., 1990).

Jane Brown (2000) has developed a model of how adolescents choose, interpret, and interact with media during their sexual development named the *Media Practice Model*. This model maintains that adolescents select and react to sexualized media because the media relate to an emerging sense of themselves as sexual beings. Using ethnographic methods, Brown suggests that what youth learn from television (e.g., soap operas), contemporary music, and other forms of media is filtered through prior knowledge and the extent to which they can identify with or imagine themselves as similar to the people being viewed or heard. Thus, what youths learn about sexuality from media depends on the media they use and the ways in which they attend to and make sense of the sexual content presented.

Television commercials use sexuality to sell products very effectively. In a study of high school girls, those who were shown commercials that use sex appeal, youth, or beauty to advertise products, in contrast to those who viewed neutral commercials, were more likely to say that beauty was important for them to feel good about themselves and to be popular with boys (Tan, 1979). Programming other than commercials also appears to influence youths' perceptions of attractiveness and beauty. For example, male students who watched a television episode of *Charlie's Angels* rated pictures of potential dates less positively than males who did not watch this program (Kenrick & Gutierres, 1980).

Other research in this area focuses on the links between soap operas and sexuality. Soap operas are a significant proportion of preadolescent and adolescent girls' television exposure. Soap opera portrayals of sexuality have been analyzed repeatedly (Brown et al., 1990; Larson, 1991). Their references to and depictions of sexual activity have increased dramatically. In soap operas popular with children and adolescents, sexual content has increased by 21% since comparable data were collected in 1982 and by 103% since 1990 (Greenberg et al., 1987). These studies also suggest that soap opera characters and storylines promote promiscuity, sexual coercion, and casual, unprotected sex (Lowry & Towles, 1989). In addition, they suggest that soap operas provide inconsistent messages concerning health-related social issues. Larson (1991) analyzed the content of the soap opera *All My Children*, a favorite of preteen and teen girls, for 1 year. Although she found that an AIDS storyline was used during that year, she noted that "AIDS was treated as a health problem for only a handful of people, not as a threat which should stimulate 'safe sex' for all. In fact, using a drug-free female [as a character with AIDS], one of the least common persons with AIDS in the U.S., diminished the authenticity of the story" (p. 162).

Although soap operas clearly present inappropriate sexual models for young viewers, other forms of mass media, such as televised films on cable networks, present even more unhealthy sexual images. Greenberg and his colleagues (1987) found that R-rated movies, seen by a majority of adolescents, contain much more frequent and more varied sexual activity than soap operas. These authors report that R-rated movies portray graphic sexual acts very often, in contrast to soap operas, which more frequently present dialogue *about* sex but actually portray sexual acts less frequently.

Another type of television programming that has been studied for its promotion of inappropriate sexual behavior is music videos (Greenfield, 1984). Content analyses of music videos that tell a story (in contrast to those that show a band playing) report that 75% of them contain sexually suggestive material and 56% contain violence that is often directed at women (Sherman & Dominick, 1986). Youthful viewers appear to be learning about sexuality from these videos. After viewing only 10 rock music videos, adolescents were more likely than those who had not viewed the videos to agree that premarital sex is acceptable (Greeson & Williams, 1986). And some of these youthful viewers appear to be more influenced by the sexuality portrayed in music videos than other youths. For example, youths who watch more music videos report more tolerant attitudes toward premarital sexual permissiveness, and are more likely than other youths to be dissatisfied with the "way things are going" in their families and more likely to consider running away from home (Strouse, Buerkel-Rothfuss, & Long, 1995). Other risky behavior may also be affected. DuRant and his colleagues (1997) found that a high percentage of music videos portray alcohol and tobacco use, particularly videos broadcast by MTV, which has an enormous youthful audience. Thus, even modest amounts of music video viewing expose children and adolescents to many portrayals of substance use. Studies suggest that the effect of music videos transcends their actual programming; when viewers hear a song after having seen the video version, they "flash back" to the visual imagery in the video (Greenfield & Beagles-Roos, 1988). In light of the huge youthful audience that these music videos attract, their potential for transmitting negative sexual images to young viewers is tremendous (Strasburger, 1992, 1995).

Music videos and soap operas present negative images of sexuality to young American viewers. However, this need not be the case, as demonstrated by the success and popular support for soap operas in Mexico and India that promote positive themes such as family planning, national integration, solution of problems of urban life, maintenance of traditional culture, and the changing status of women. Young viewers who have the opportunity to see aspects of responsible sexuality such as contraceptive use and HIV prevention discussions by sexually active couples on their favorite programs may more easily incorporate such behavior into their own sexual scripts.

Many questions concerning these effects are unanswered. These issues include the effects of viewing this programming with same-sex or opposite-sex peers, the extent to which young viewers believe that television is a credible source of sexual information, and the developmental impact of sexual television programming on sexuality (Greenberg et al., 1987).

Other Negative Health Consequences of Media Use

The harmful health effects of children's media use is dramatized by the convulsion and seizure activity documented in some children while watching TV or using electronic games. On December 16, 1997, about 700 children across Japan were hospitalized because of convulsive seizures or vomiting experienced while watching the Pokemon program on television (Kobayashi, Takayama, Mihara, & Sugishita, 1999). Research and clinical studies since then have reported many neurological problems in children during photic stimulation such as that experienced while playing Pokemon or watching it on TV. Furusho and colleagues (1998) documented this seizure activity. A survey of 662 children and their parents revealed that most of them (603, 91%) had watched the program, and 30 of the children reported associated neuropsychological abnormalities including seizures, headaches, nausea and vomiting, blurred vision, and vertigo. Another study, conducted in Europe, deliberately exposed children with histories of photosensitivity to provocative series of intermittent photic, patterned televised stimulants, including standard television programming and Super Mario World (Kasteleijn-Nolst, Trenite et al., 1999). More of these children demonstrated neuropsychological sensitivity when playing Super Mario World than when watching standard television programs. Further research suggests that most serious seizures occur during Pokemon and other program scenes in which red and blue frames alternate at the rate of 12 flashes per second; the incidence of such induced seizures appears to be about 1 in 5,000 children aged 6–18 years (Kobayashi et al., 1999; Takada et al., 1999).

Other potentially detrimental, even lethal, influences of television on children's health have also been investigated. The role of watching television and playing TV-connected video games (with their exposure to magnetic fields) in contracting childhood leukemia has been investigated (Kaune et al. 2000). No evidence of a causal relationship was found.

Television sets, as heavy electrical appliances, have been implicated in a deadly way in children's environments. Retrospective analysis of files compiled by the U.S. Consumer Product Safety Commission reveal 73 cases of pediatric injuries from falling television sets, including those resulting in 28 child deaths (Bernard, Johnston, Curtis, & King, 1998). These TVs fell most often on the head, accounting for 72 of these injuries. The vast majority of the injuries involved televisions that were being supported by dressers or TV stands. These findings suggest that children can be protected from these injuries with safer, more secure locations and safer designs of support furniture.

A variety of other pediatric maladies and injuries may result from watching television. Television-viewing habits have been linked to sleep disturbances in school-age children (Owens et al., 1999). A study of almost 500 children between the ages of 5 and 10 years examined child and family television-watching patterns and a variety of child sleep behaviors including bedtime resistance, sleep onset delay, sleep duration, anxiety about sleep, parasomnia, nighttime waking, and daytime sleepiness. Results indicated that watching a lot of television daily and watching it at bedtime were related to greater sleep disturbance, particularly for those children (about 25%) who had a television set in their own bedrooms. The domains most affected were bedtime resistance, sleep onset delay, anxiety about sleep, and shortened sleep duration. The presence of a television set in a child's bedroom may be a relatively unrecognized but important contributor to schoolchildren's sleep problems.

Another problem is childhood back pain attributed to electronic media use. School physicians performed a lumbar spine examination on 392 Belgian 9-year-old children. Almost half of them had experienced at least one episode of lower back pain (Gunzburg et al., 1999). Significantly more of these children, compared to children who had not experienced even one episode of lower back pain, reported playing video games for more than 2 hours per day. However, there was no such relation for the number of hours of television watching.

Television and Suicide

Over the past three decades, youth suicide rates have increased fourfold, explaining 8% of all youth mortality (Strasburger, 1995). A few studies have documented the relation between television watching and child and youth suicide (Mishara, 1999; Phillips, Carstensen, & Paight, 1989). These studies – based on the hypothesis that attractive models of suicidal behavior, portrayed in a realistic manner, and ignoring the negative aspects of suicide including suffering and dying – suggest that certain young viewers are more susceptible than others to imitating the behavior of television programs or news reports focused on suicide. For example, one study in New York City examined both attempted and completed suicides for youth following the televising of four movies offering suicidal models over several months (Gould & Shaffer, 1989). Results demonstrated that, controlling for other variables, the average number of children's suicide attempts and completions in the 2-week period following the broadcast of these movies was much greater than the average number in the 2 weeks before the telecasts. This finding is typical of those found in investigations of suicidal behavior following the televising of a fictional suicide. In fact, there has been a significant increase in youth suicides in Western countries since the mid-1980s. This may be accounted for by Haefner and Schmidtke's (1989) hypothesis that these suicides are consequences of the expansion of the mass media and its increasing tolerance of attractive models of self-destructive behavior.

Strasburger (1992) argues that the glorification of guns on American television contributes to youthful suicide as well, in light of the facts that the presence of a gun in a household is one of the strongest predictors of adolescent suicide (Christoffel & Christoffel, 1986; Schetky, 1985) and that over 44% of children aged 6–12 years report having a gun in their home (American Health Foundation, 1995). In sum, television viewing may not simply lead to poor health habits or inappropriate sexual practices. For a vulnerable group of adolescents, it may even increase the suicide rate.

Final Thoughts on Television and Children's Health

Television is an effective and efficient teacher of many health attitudes and behaviors, both positive and negative. Although television has immense potential for creating a positive health orientation in children, currently it does not do so. Content analyses of health-relevant television programming suggest that models of health-deleterious and risky behavior far outnumber models of health-promoting behavior. When television stars risk their health and safety, entertainment potential is maximized; by contrast, television reminders of healthy and safe behaviors are presented minimally or in a less captivating fashion (Potts et al., 1996). However, television can be a significant source of pro-health messages. In a content analysis of prime-time televised news, pediatric health news was featured in 21% of national medical news stories and concentrated on nutrition (30%), allergies (21%), and major illnesses (21%). But these clips are often not designed to attract children's attention; instead, they are largely aimed at adults. Almost two-thirds of the parents surveyed and about one-half of the pediatricians surveyed in this study believed that television reports are important sources of child health information (Prabhu, Duffy, & Stapleton, 1996).

Parental management of children's television viewing can be a potentially positive socialization influence in other ways as well (Huston & Wright, 1996, 1998; Levin, 1998; Valerio, Amodio, Dalzio, Vianello, & Zacchello, 1997). Parents can modify the effects of children's television viewing by watching television with children, and by acting as positive models of television use and decision making about the quality and quantity of television viewing. Much of children's media use is unsupervised by parents (Roberts, 2000). However, as noted earlier in this chapter, parental viewing of television with children has been proposed as a means of increasing the positive messages gained by children (Carlson et al., 1996; St. Peters et al., 1991). Coviewing changes developmentally. Studies indicate that kindergarten children view television with others about 85% of the time: with mothers (27%), fathers (18%), and older siblings (62%) (Field, 1987). However, for elementary schoolchildren, between one-half and two-thirds of coviewing is with parents. Other studies suggest that these data are more ambiguous than they seem. Some researchers report higher rates of coviewing for older children (6th and 10th graders) than for younger children (2nd graders) (Dorr, Kovaric, & Doubleday, 1989), whereas others have found that younger children view programs with their parents more frequently than do older children (St. Peters et al., 1991). In spite of the uncertainty concerning the developmental trends in coviewing, these is little question about the importance of this shared activity for children. Television viewing accounts for a substantial amount of shared family activity. One of the advantages of children coviewing with more cognitively sophisticated individuals, such as parents, is the opportunity to improve children's comprehension of the content as the older viewer comments on the action and message of the program (Huston & Wright, 1996). Media literacy, the art of deconstructing television for children, gives parents an opportunity to discuss values, beliefs, and moral issues (Messaris & Sarett, 1981). If a program includes such events, parents can explain to children that television programs exist to deliver audiences to advertisers, that sex and violence sell advertisers' products, and that television news and entertainment programming is designed to get the best ratings. Unless parents are confident that a television program does not contain unwanted material, parents can watch with their children and talk to them about controversial content. Parents can ask their older children such questions as "When that character decided to have sex with a man she just met at a party, wouldn't it have been wise for her to insist that he wear a condom?" or "How can women effectively suggest that men use condoms when having sex?" Although children cannot be effectively "immunized" against all inappropriate and misleading television content, these methods can help parents give children information in an informal setting about hard-to-discuss topics, such as sexuality, and correct casual and irresponsible televised messages about health-related behavior to which children are regularly exposed. Furthermore, parents' ultimate goal in regulating and participating in their children's television viewing is to encourage children to develop their own self-monitoring abilities, so that as they develop, they will become increasingly competent and savvy in choosing and deconstructing televised programming for themselves (Kubey, 1986).

Television is ubiquitous in our society and an inescapable element in most children's lives. As eminent television researchers Aletha Huston and John Wright so eloquently remind us: "the family is the core socializing force influencing children's use of television and what they learn from it. Most television is viewed at home. Children's early exposure to television occurs largely through the viewing choices of . . . families, and viewing is often a family affair" (1996, p. 39). It is critical for families to harness this powerful influence for promotion of children's health and prevention of harm.

8

The Social Ecology of Children's Health Socialization

Children's health attitudes, behavior, and health status are affected by the environment in which children are reared. This environment enables or constrains child health behavior and status (Richter et al., 2000). Some aspects of this perspective on children's health have been researched; others have not. My examination of this research focuses on three issues: socioeconomic status, families' impact on the emotional climate of children's lives, and the impact of parents' health on children's health.

Socioeconomic Status

Demographic status, specifically socioeconomic status, has traditionally been the focus of efforts to describe and predict children's health (American Academy of Pediatrics, 2000a; DiLiberti, 2000; Hertzman, 1999). However, social class is not an explanatory variable, and in most cases it merely describes parents and children who vary in health attitudes, behavior, and actual health. In this book, in contrast to its traditional use, social class is conceptualized as a proxy for a broad set of environmental characteristics that may be associated with children's health socialization in health-enhancing or health-constraining conditions.

Recent statistics indicate that more children in the United States are living in poverty than in any recent period. More than one-quarter of American children under age 6 are living in poverty, although nearly three in five poor children have working parents (National Center for Children in Poverty, 1995). Adults and children of higher social class usually have access to better health services, use them more frequently, and have better health (Adler et al., 1994; Aylward, 1992). Parental socioeconomic variables such as age, education, occupation, and income are aspects of socioeconomic status associated with children's health status. These factors appear to strongly influence the health environment in which children develop by modifying such aspects as parent–child interaction (e.g., maternal teaching strategies, disciplinary tactics), parental beliefs and attitudes, physical attributes (space, crowding, cleanliness, noise), organization, regularity and predictability of schedules and caregiving, and the availability of food, materials, and other resources. Several researchers have investigated the relation between environment and health, most notably Sameroff (Sameroff, 1998; Sameroff & Chandler, 1975; Sameroff, Seifer, Zaks, & Barocas, 1987). Results of these studies confirm that single environmental risk factors have smaller effects on health and development but that the accumulation of risk factors produces geometric increases in childhood morbidity (Aylward, 1992). Moreover, the transactional model of Sameroff and Chandler (1975) suggests that children are constantly reorganizing adaptively in the context of their environment. Poor environments compromise children's developmental progress, while more favorable environments promote childhood resilience and better outcomes.

Other related research suggests an association between physical and social disadvantage during childhood and lifetime exposure to health-damaging environments. Occupational, residential, and household histories were used to generate lifetime exposures to a range of environmental hazards for almost 300 adults. These histories were related to the findings of clinical physical examinations of the participants at ages 5–14 years (Holland et al., 2000). Results indicated significant relations between their lifetime exposure to health-damaging environments and physical health indicators in childhood. For example, age-adjusted height during childhood was found to be inversely related to subsequent exposure to hazards for males whose fathers had manual occupations and for females whose fathers had nonmanual occupations. Chronic disease during childhood was also associated with greater subsequent hazard exposure in males with fathers who had manual jobs. However, for females whose fathers had nonmanual jobs, chronic disease during childhood was related to reduced subsequent hazard exposure. The authors of this report suggest that exposure to health-damaging environments during adulthood may be added to health disadvantage during childhood, and that this process of life course accumulation of disadvantage may vary by gender and childhood social class (Holland et al., 2000).

Children learn about health during their interactions with their parents, who are in most cases their primary socialization agents during infancy and early childhood. Therefore, from this perspective, the role the parents play in structuring and maintaining a health-enhancing or health-deleterious environment for their child, as a function of their socioeconomic status, is a focus of parents' impact on children's health (Fiese & Sameroff, 1989).

Studies demonstrate that although childhood mortality has declined in recent decades in all social classes in the United States (although less so in children of lower-class parents), childhood morbidity remains dispro-portionately high in children in lower socioeconomic groups. Utilization of childhood preventive and ameliorative health services, as well as child-hood morbidity, is not distributed randomly; a number of studies have shown that parents living in environments characterized by high levels of stress and low levels of support are poor utilizers of health services, espe-cially well-child services (Children's Defense Fund, 1988). Low-income parents take their children to pediatricians or primary care providers, den-tists, and immunization providers less often than higher-income parents (Rosenstock & Kirscht, 1980). Even when health services are designed specifically for low-income families, those parents within low-income groups with more education and nontargeted parents who normally use services utilize the services more often than targeted low-income parents with less education (Elinson, Henshaw, & Cohen, 1976).

As this study demonstrates, education, as one of the most significant aspects of social class, has a powerful effect on how children learn to take care of their health. This is further exemplified by a study by Hupkens and colleagues (Hupkens, Knibbe, Van Otterloo, & Drop, 1998). Using education as a classifying variable, these researchers examined the impact of social class on mothers' imposition of food rules on their children to determine whether more-educated mothers prescribe more healthy foods and restrict more unhealthy foods for their children than less-educated mothers. This study also investigated whether mothers with more educa-tion considered health aspects more often and the preferences of their children less often in choosing food for their children than mothers with less education. Mothers of young children were asked about their food practices. Results demonstrated that all mothers prescribed foods such as meat and vegetables for their children's dinners. Most mothers limited their children's consumption of sweets, soft drinks, and snacks. Mothers with more education restricted more foods than mothers with less educa-tion, but there were no effects of education level on the food items they prescribed for their children.

Research on social class and children's health finds that lower socio-economic status is related to less knowledge about health, less positive health-related attitudes, less stoicism when ill, and less healthy lifestyle practices in both parents and children (Auslander, Haire-Joshu, Rogge, & Santiago, 1991; Donovan, Jessor, & Costa, 1991; Sigelman et al., 1993). Specific illnesses such as asthma, gastroenteritis, influenza, meningitis, otitis media, respiratory infections, and rheumatic fever are found more frequently in children from lower socioeconomic groups even when ethnicity is statistically controlled for (Butler, Starfield, & Stenmark, 1984; Margolis, Keyes, Greenberg, Bauman, & LaVange, 1997; Vignerova et al., 2000). Children from lower socioeconomic groups have more restricted activity days, miss more school days, are more often confined to bed, are more overweight, experience more unintentional injuries, and spend two to four times as many days hospitalized as children from the middle and upper classes (Egbuonu & Starfield, 1982; Reading, Langford, Haynes, & Lovett, 1999). In fact, socioeconomic status has been identified as the single best predictor of child health, even controlling for ethnicity and other related variables (Morse, Hyde, Newberger, & Reed, 1977; Schaefer, 1979). However, as noted previously, socioeconomic status is a descriptive rather than an explanatory variable, and also covaries with several factors known to influence health behavior, including family structure and income and parental education, which appear to be strongly related to utilization of childhood health services and child health. For example, several papers from the National Health Examination Survey examined the utility of various family demographic variables as predictors of child health (Edwards & Grossman, 1978, 1979; Shakato, Edwards, & Grossman, 1980). The results of these studies suggested that parents' education, especially that of the mother, was the best predictor of child health status. Results from a study of children's conceptions of health as a function of varying socioeconomic environments suggests additional mechanisms of these relations (Normandeau, Kalnins, Jutras, & Hanigan, 1998). Over 1,500 children aged 5–12 years from different rural and urban living environments were interviewed concerning various aspects of health: criteria of good health, behaviors necessary to maintain health, consequences of being healthy, and health threats. Depending on the socioeconomic status of their families, children demonstrated a complex understanding of health that could be organized by three dimensions: being functional, adhering to good lifestyle health behaviors, and mental health (i.e., a general sense of well-being and good relationships with others).

Children of single mothers fare poorly on a number of indicators of physical well-being, and it appears that socioeconomic status is an underlying factor in this linkage (Cooper & Weinick, 1999; Heck & Parker,

1999). For example, in a study of over 63,000 children less than 18 years of age in the National Health Interview Surveys of 1993–1995, family structure and access to health care differed by maternal education. Although children of mothers with 16 or more years of education had greater access to care overall, increasing maternal education was associated with relatively less access to care for children of single mothers compared with children in two-parent families. Thus, children of single mothers were at a relative disadvantage with respect to health care compared to children in two-parent families only at higher levels of maternal education (Heck & Parker, 1999).

Gender Influences on Health as a Function of Children's Social Class

Children's gender appears to affect the relations between children's health and social class. Analyses of health data on a sample of over 60,000 Finnish children indicated that boys had greater overall health risk than girls. However, gender differences in health indicators that are more social class–based (e.g., risk of delayed development, postponed school start, attendance in special education programs) were substantially greater than those for more biologically based child health indicators (Gissler, Jarvelink, Louhiala, & Hemminki, 1999). Results from another study complicate this picture even further, suggesting gender by ethnicity by social class interaction effects. Jackson and colleagues (Jackson, Treiber, Turner, Davis, & Strong, 1999) examined children's cardiovascular responsivity to and recovery from acute laboratory stressors during and after a variety of tasks (e.g., video game playing, interview, parent–child conflict discussion). African American children had higher blood pressure and lower heart rate responsivity than Euro-American children. However, an ethnicity by social class interaction for systolic blood pressure was found in which lower-class Euro-American and higher-class African American children had the greatest responsivity compared to their same-ethnicity cohorts. In recovery, African American children and all male children exhibited higher systolic blood pressure than Euro-American and female children.

Finally, relevant to children's gender influences on the relations between social class and children's health is a study of adult health status based on childhood social class compared across gender. Utilizing longitudinal data from the cohort of English people born in 1958, researchers found no gender differences in health as a function of childhood social class. However, gender differences in health based on a specific aspect of childhood social class – education – were found among men in this sample at age 33 with respect to chronic illness and respiratory symptoms. Men at age 33 who grew up in lower-class homes experienced more chronic illness and respiratory symptoms than did men of the same age who were raised in middle-class homes. Women who were raised in lower-class families experienced poorer health and more psychological stress at age 23 than women who grew up in middle-class homes. Thus, these results suggest gender differences in health as a function of childhood social class that are inconsistent across age and type of health indicator (Matthews, Manor, & Power, 1999).

Socioeconomic status can affect other aspects of children's health as well. Zero Population Growth ranked 828 U.S. cities using 70 population-related social, economic, and environmental indicators that affect children's risk, and found that in many geographic areas children are under a great deal of stress. Sources of stress affecting health to which lower-class children were particularly vulnerable included many residential moves, overcrowding, crime, maternal unemployment, and environmental degradation (Zero Population Growth, 1993). For example, frequent residential moves can contribute to children's health risk in the following way. All calls in several months of 1986–1987 to the Central Virginia Poison Control Center regarding the ingestion of poison by children younger than 6 years of age were systematically studied (Garretson, Bush, Gates, & French, 1990). The results suggested that half of all the poisoning incidents involved substances that had been moved, used, or placed such that they were unusually accessible and perhaps likely to attract the attention of the child on the day the incident occurred. In fact, nearly one-fourth of all the poisoning incidents occurred within 1 hour of the change in the poison environment. Poisonous substances are often moved from their original storage location when families move; therefore, poor families who must frequently move put their children at risk in a unique and probably unrecognized way. A second way in which residential relocation can affect children's health was noted by Fowler and her associates (Fowler, Simpson, & Schoendorf, 1993). In analyses of data from the National Health Interview Survey of Child Health, demographic and mobility information on 17,110 children and their families was studied. The results suggest that children whose families move frequently are at risk in another health-related manner. Whereas across the United States about 8% of children do not have a regular provider for preventive health services, 7% do not have a regular provider of sick care, and 3% regularly utilize an emergency room for sick care, these percentages are much higher for children whose families had moved three or more times in the child's lifetime. Of these children, 14% lacked a regular provider for preventive care and 10% did not have a regular provider for sick care. Children who had moved more than twice were 3.0 times as likely to lack a regular provider for preventive or sick care and 1.6 times as likely to use an emergency room for sick care as were children who never moved. Thus, families who move often are less likely to have access to regular providers for their children's preventive or sick care and more likely to use emergency room services when their children are sick. Together, these studies highlight just two of the ways in which the geographical locations (and change in locations) in which parents raise their children can contribute to the childhood health risk.

Familial stress itself has been related to negative health outcomes (O'Leary, 1990), and in addition has been demonstrated to mediate other factors that can themselves lead to poorer health outcomes. For example, Henggeler and his colleagues (1991) found that high levels of television viewing among children, which is associated with exercise and nutritional deficits in childhood, is linked with maternal reports of high family stress. Stress associated with negative family life events has been demonstrated to result in sleeping and waking problems in childhood, which in turn is related to more physical and mental health problems (Tobia, Wolfson, & Gallagher, 1995). Several researchers have noted that recurrent abdominal pain (RAP) in childhood appears to be the direct result of exposure to psychological stress, individual differences in reacting to stress, and maladaptive ways of coping with stress (Baeyer & Walker, 1999; Compas & Harding Thomsen, 1999). The mechanism of these relations is hypothesized in two different but related ways. Exposure to stress may precipitate RAP. Alternatively, both acute and chronic stress contribute to increases in central nervous system arousal, which in turn may lead to gastrointestinal dysfunction (Compas & Harding Thomsen, 1999).

The Impact of Parent–Child Emotional Interactions on Children's Health

Some research has examined the relations between emotional family process variables and children's health. This research is based on the concept of the family as the "breeding ground for somatic complaints" (Fiese & Sameroff, 1989, p. 294). For example, Minuchin (1985) described how children's physical symptoms can be related to family interactions characterized as enmeshed, overprotective, and rigid. Walker and Greene

(1987) demonstrated that children whose families have low cohesion report more physical symptoms than those with high family cohesion. In our study of preschool children and their parents (Lees & Tinsley, 1998), various characteristics of children's family dynamics were significantly related to mothers' and teachers' reports of children's health behavior. For example, more family cohesion was associated with children's independent compliance with regular bedtimes. Perhaps children in cohesive families feel particularly motivated to comply with household health rules. Another finding from this study was that as reports of family conflict increase, mothers state that children select nutritious snacks and use seat belts less often. These findings might be explained as a function of parental energy in conflicted families; perhaps family energy is being spent on conflict and not on teaching children independence or responsibility for behavior. Or it is possible that the child's contentiousness about the use of a seat belt is one source of family conflict (Tinsley et al., 2002). One child behavior, selecting healthy food often, is related to two somewhat associated family characteristics: a moral-religious emphasis in the family and the use of control as a method of system maintenance. Perhaps children in families with these characteristics select healthy foods to maintain order by "doing the right thing." Thus, it appears that family interaction and dynamics characteristics are associated with children's health-related behavior, as measured independently by teachers and mothers. Again, the mechanisms of this association are unexplored, but they provide fruitful areas for future research on the development of children's health behavior in the family context.

Another area of inquiry focused on the links between parent–child interaction and children's health is the quality of parent–child relationships in relation to children's health status. In spite of the fact that the parent–child relationship is affectively laden, until quite recently the recognition of an emotional component to child socialization has been conspicuously missing from the child preventive health literature. Emotion is a primary component of parent and child attentional, motivational, and goal development processes (Ratner & Stettner, 1991). Affect can explain individual differences in how children and parents respond to various situations, their causal attributions, and the manner in which they construct and interpret situations (Dix & Reinhold, 1991; Dodge, 1991; MacKinnon, Lamb, Belsky, & Baum, 1990). Thus, a discussion of children's health socialization must acknowledge the importance of affective processes. Parents' and children's emotions play an important role in health and illness care, and in teaching and learning healthy behaviors and attitudes, and generally influence all aspects of parent–child health socialization interactions. Some evidence appears to confirm these suppositions. Measures of parent–child attachment security are related to symptom reporting, health care utilization, and restriction of normal activities (Feeney, 2000). These links appear to be explained, at least in part, by individual differences in emotional and behavioral response to stress, with physiological and biochemical pathways explaining some of the effects of attachment style on children's physical health. The quality of parent–child attachment also predicts family responses to children's illness, as reflected in parents' visitation rates and family participation during child hospitalization (Feeney, 2000).

Parmelee (1986, 1992) noted that parents feel a strong responsibility to keep their children healthy. The minor illnesses that children are certain to encounter during their early years may serve as an indictment of parents' caregiving abilities, causing feelings of uncertainty and inadequacy. Thus, the protection of children's healthy status is an emotionally charged issue for parents. In addition, successful management of children's illnesses can help parents develop self-confidence (Parmelee, 1986, 1992). Effectively teaching children healthful and preventive behaviors would also be expected to validate parental self-confidence and positive affect. Thus, emotion is a potent component of parent–child interactions as parents protect their children's health, successfully manage their illnesses, and effectively teach their children to take over their own health care (Tinsley & Lees, 1995).

Emotional Processes during Health Teaching

Although previous chapters of this book have examined the effects of parents' cognitions on processes of health socialization, these thoughts and attributions were primarily discussed as if they were independent of any influence of emotion. However, to fully understand the influence of parents' cognitions during the socialization of certain health tasks, it is also essential to examine how emotion intervenes in the process. Emotional processes have a variety of roles during parents' attempts to teach their children health behaviors. For example, Ratner and Stettner (1991) suggest that shared affect leads to shared understanding between parent and child, and that this shared understanding is necessary for internalization and learning to occur.

Emotion impels all steps of the teaching and learning processes. Parental emotion highlights certain aspects of the situation, gaining the child's attention; reciprocally, the child's attentional processes are delimited by her emotional state and involvement. Parents' affective responses can also help maintain or interfere with the child's interest and attention and can emphasize the important aspects of the transaction – for example, by facial or verbal expression or emphasis – whereas the child's affect indicates to his parent what aspects of the event are more or less interesting.

Diaz, Neal, and Vachio (1991) found that parents motivate their children to take over responsibility for tasks by creating positive, nurturing environments for learning experiences. Because warm teaching interactions have been demonstrated to increase children's autonomous and self-regulated performance, children's compliance in joint learning is increased, and children are more likely to internalize control and ultimately comply even during adult absence (Diaz et al., 1991). Thus, positive parental affect while teaching children to care for their health increases the effectiveness of socialization – that is, children will be more competent and independent in self-care. Finally, parental affect in response to children's errors influences their ensuing emotional and cognitive responses (Ratner & Stettner, 1991). For example, whereas a child whose mother became angry when he was unable to perform an expected task independently might experience negative affect – frustration or sadness – a child whose parent was patient and encouraging, under the same circumstances, might be more positive and inspired to work harder to master the same task (Tinsley & Lees, 1995).

The relative salience of cognitive and emotional components varies in different socialization experiences. For example, when parents teach a child to place a correct puzzle piece, the cognitive element is probably much more pronounced than the affective one. However, because of parents' strong motivation to keep their children healthy and teach them important health behaviors (Parmelee, 1986, 1992, 1997), emotional factors would be expected to be much more salient during health or safety socialization. Thus, parents might express high affect when insisting that a child fasten her seat belt every time they ride in a car, and many parents are extremely forceful when encouraging their young children to finish their vegetables before ending the meal. In addition, even within the health socialization context, variability in the emotional content of these interactions would be expected. For example, a parent teaching a child to squeeze toothpaste onto a toothbrush would not demonstrate the same affective involvement as one teaching a preschooler to always wash and disinfect a cut. On the other hand, children who are restrained from a desired goal – such as eating candy – may experience more affective involvement than when learning to wash their hands after using the toilet (Lees & Tinsley, 1998).

The preceding examples should not suggest that emotion and cognition are orthogonal aspects of child socialization. When examining the effect of parental attributions of children's behaviors on parental emotional responses, Dix demonstrated clear connections between emotions and cognition (Dix & Grusec, 1983; Dix & Reinhold, 1991). Dix and his associates found that whereas emotional states, such as mood, influence parental attributions about their children's responsibility for negative behaviors, parental cognitions, both about situational factors and about their stable childrearing ideologies, also modify their emotional responses to their child's behaviors. These findings demonstrate an interactive influence of emotion and cognition on parental responses to children. Thus, the affective and cognitive components of experience cannot be separated. Parents and children construct interpretations of an event, and of each other's behaviors and motivations, that influence ensuing interactions and behaviors (MacKinnon et al., 1990). Thus, when interpreting parental socialization of children's health behaviors and attitudes, emotion and cognition must be examined together (Lees & Tinsley, 1998).

Emotion as an Integral Part of Health Contexts

In the course of childhood health socialization, both the emotional and the behavioral nature of experience are socialized. Emotion provides a context for understanding situations and producing behaviors. In addition, affect constrains all aspects of information processing. Researchers who study parent–child attachment relationships have noted that individuals are prone to remember affectively salient experiences and that they form schemas – *internal working models* (Ainsworth, Blehar, Waters, & Wall, 1978) or *emotion dispositions* (MacKinnon et al., 1990) – of these events that become frameworks and constraints for their behaviors in, understanding of, and interpretation of future experiences (Main, Kaplan, & Cassidy, 1985; Sroufe & Fleeson, 1986). These theorists suggest that even when the affect associated with an experience is negative or unpleasant, individuals often seek out or create experiences similar to familiar ones in order to maintain consistency and control over their world (MacKinnon et al., 1990). Within the health context, experiences are frequently emotionally laden. Illness, doctor visits, and medical procedures and immunizations, for example, are often quite emotional experiences for children. In addition, emotion is often strongly identified with some health (or unhealthy) behaviors such as eating sweets for comfort or engaging in risky behaviors when distressed. For example, when food is often used as a comforting device or as a reward, the act of eating may eventually be associated with positive affect, resulting in overeating. These emotion-bound behavior patterns often originate within the family during childhood (Tinsley & Lees, 1995).

Dodge (1991) proposed that emotion has an important role in social information processing. He suggested that emotion influences this process in four ways: (1) as an arousal state, (2) in goal setting, (3) in the experience of emotion, and (4) as expressive behavior. The role of emotion as an arousal state that influences parents' and children's attentional processes has been discussed. Parents and children use emotional cues and responses to draw and maintain each other's attention. An extremely low level of emotional arousal might result in reduced attention on the part of the child and decreased learning. Alternatively, heightened arousal caused by emotion has been found to have a negative effect on cue interpretation, which can influence the accuracy of one's interpretation of an experience. For example, overaroused boys tend to overattribute hostile intentions to peers (Dodge, 1991; Dodge & Somberg, 1987).

Emotion is an important component of goal setting in two ways: Emotional goals, rather than health-oriented goals, may motivate health behavior, and the emotional nature of conflicting goals may result in individuals choosing to take risks with their health. Individuals frequently choose and pursue goals for emotional rather than cognitive or rational reasons. In addition, goals are not always manifest in observable behavior. Children (and adults) often perform health behaviors in the pursuit of goals that are not at all health oriented. For example, at 13 years of age, a boy often starts to bathe, wash his hair, and brush his teeth daily without being reminded. Whereas his parents might be tempted to interpret this behavior as resulting from his maturing understanding of the relation between cleanliness and health, his actual reason may be his enhanced, and highly emotional, interest in being attractive to 13-year-old girls. Similarly, parents who take a 5-year-old to the doctor for a checkup and immunizations solely to fulfill kindergarten entry requirements are obtaining health care for their child for reasons not entirely related to health motivations. In these situations, health behaviors, impelled by apparently health-oriented goals, often have purposes somewhat remote from health enhancement, even though health improvement may result. In this manner, an unrelated emotional objective ultimately results in health behavior (Tinsley & Lees, 1995).

Dodge (1991) also suggested that some children may be more adversely affected by the same emotional conditions. He described these children as "emotionally vulnerable" and indicated that they were more disregulated – cognitively disrupted – by emotional states than were other children. Dodge and Somberg (1987) demonstrated this emotional vulnerability in aggressive boys. They found that when aggressive and non-aggressive boys were exposed to an emotionally negative experience, the aggressive boys made more errors in interpreting the intentions of others and exhibited a hostile attributional bias when emotionally aroused. This indicates that some children are more sensitive, and vulnerable, to upsetting experiences. It also explains individual differences in children's reactions to emotional medical events such as doctor visits or illness, which for some are extremely negative experiences, whereas others take them in stride. However, although attributional bias may explain how some of these individual differences operate, it does not demonstrate how these differences evolve. Dodge (1991) proposed a mechanism having to do with past negative affective experiences and reactions that must be further examined in future studies. Although the mechanism of these effects is yet to be fully determined, Dodge's arguments and investigations clearly indicate an important role of emotion and emotional sensitivity in the socialization of children's health and illness behaviors and feelings.

When parents socialize children, they socialize the appropriate emotional responses in addition to the correct behaviors. As children grow, and take more responsibility for health and safety tasks, they become responsible for both the cognitive and emotional components of these behaviors. Warton and Goodnow (1991) suggested that as children mature and take over responsibility for task performance, there is also a transfer of responsibility for the emotional content of the experience. For example, when a very young child is not clean, the parent is embarrassed. However, as children get older, they are expected to take over both the responsibility for and the emotion of the event. Therefore, a young teen would be expected to take care of his or her own cleanliness and should feel uncomfortable or embarrassed when he or she is not clean (Lees & Tinsley, 1998).

Affect influences all aspects of parent–child interactions. It impacts attention, goal setting, event interpretation, and responses; it influences attributions about others' behavior; and it even impacts on the reactions of others. In addition, health provides a context that is replete with emotional content. Thus, the socialization of children's health behaviors cannot be understood without recognizing and examining their behavioral, cognitive, and emotional components (Wood, Klebba, & Miller, 2000).

O'Leary (1990), in an in-depth review of the relations between stress, emotion, and immune function, suggests that emotional experience, including affect regulation, appears to be an immunologic mediator of health. One such indicator of emotional experience, mother–child attachment quality, appears to affect children's health (Feeney, 2000). Early family experiences of illness, mother–child attachment style (secure, avoidant, anxious/ambivalent), and three health outcomes (symptom reporting, health services utilization, and health status) were assessed in a sample of college freshmen (Feeney & Ryan, 1994). Findings confirmed that parent–child attachment style was related to maternal responses to subjects' early childhood illness. Specifically, avoidant attachment was negatively related to parental overindulgence during childhood illness and negatively related to parental responsiveness. Anxious/ambivalent attachment was positively related to reported parental overindulgence, and avoidant attachment was inversely linked with later visits to health care professionals. The results of this study suggest important implications for the influence of parent–child relationships on physical well-being, and specifically highlight the relation between child affect regulation, as a function of parent–child interaction, and later health behavior and outcomes.

One set of physical health effects of a disrupted emotional climate in families with very young children has been identified and documented: failure to thrive (Drotar & Robinson, 2000). The term *failure to thrive* is used to diagnose children, often infants, who are underweight or malnourished. Some children experience failure to thrive because of an illness or a medical disorder. However, sometimes growth failure is due to environmental neglect or social stimulus deprivation. In many of these cases, the psychological basis of failure to thrive appears similar to that of hospitalism, a syndrome observed in babies who have depression secondary to being understimulated. The unstimulated child becomes depressed, apathetic, and ultimately anorexic. Stimulation may be lacking because the caregiver (usually the mother) is herself depressed or apathetic, has poor parenting skills, is anxious about or unfulfilled by the caregiving role, feels hostile toward the child, or is responding to real or perceived external stresses (e.g., demands of other children in large or chaotic families, marital instability, a significant personal loss, financial difficulties). However, poor caregiving by the mother does not fully account for this type of failure to thrive. The child's temperament, capacities, and responses help shape maternal nurturance patterns, and failure to thrive may be considered the result of dysfunctional interactions between caregiver and child. These cases can also be characterized as a caregiver–child mismatch in which the child's demands, although not pathological, cannot be adequately met by the caregiver, who might, however, do well with a child who has different needs or even with the same child under different circumstances. Treatment consists of providing education and emotional support to correct the problems interfering with the caregiver–child relationship.

A related avenue of research has considered the impact of parental anxiety on children's health behavior and health status. Three effects of parental anxiety on child health behavior and health status have been identified: the effects on the child's behavior during medical procedures, on utilization of health care services, and on minor illness in childhood.

In a study of children's fear and coping during medical examinations, Bush, Melamed, Sheras, and Greenbaum (1986) found that high maternal state and trait anxiety was related to poor ratings of children's handling of previous medical experiences. Additionally, mothers who were agitated provided less information and ignored their children more. The authors suggested that maternal anxiety is associated with patterns of mothering during medical events characterized by less effectiveness and more disorganization.

Consistent with earlier research in this area (Campion & Gabriel, 1985; Roghmann, Hecht, & Haggerty, 1973), Goldman and Owen (1994), in an investigation of the relation between maternal trait anxiety and mothers' utilization of pediatric services for their infants, found that mothers' reports of anxiety during pregnancy predicted increased use of pediatric acute care visits during infancy. In interpreting these results, Goldman and Owen suggest that highly anxious mothers may be hypervigilant for health problems in their children and more predisposed to consult formal health institutions to determine their etiology. These findings become even more interesting when considered in light of data from Richtsmeier and Hatcher (1994) suggesting that highly anxious parents appear to have a poorer understanding of their children's condition following their interaction with a pediatrician. Together, these studies suggest that parental anxiety about children's health has many negative influences on children's health behavior and status.

The Impact of Parents' Interactions with Others on Children's Health

Another way in which parents influence their children's health is through the effect of their interactions with others, especially other family members. A series of studies by Cummings and his colleagues (Cummings,

1998; Cummings, Goeke-Morey, & Dukewich, 2001), Gottman and his associates (Gottman & Katz, 1989; Hooven, Gottman, & Katz, 1995), as well as a review by Grych and Fincham (1990), suggest that children's exposure to parent–parent anger and hostility is a source of physiological stress for children. Cummings et al. (2001) suggest that children's responses to familial background anger include physiological responses. Cummings (1998) and Cummings et al. (2001) also suggest that whether or not children have the opportunity to determine if background anger has been resolved can affect children's emotional and physiological responses. Viewing hostile disagreements was reported by children to be the most negative and elicited the most anger in children. Unresolved background anger was perceived by children as more negative and resulted in more hostile reactions in children (Cummings, 1998; Cummings et al., 2001).

Two studies by Gottman and his colleagues suggest that the way parents manage their emotions in dealing with each other may have striking effects on their children's physical health. The first study investigated the effects of marital discord on the physical health of preschool children (Gottman & Katz, 1989). Results suggested direct and indirect pathways by which parent marital upset interferes with children's social development, which in turn increases children's susceptibility to illness. Specifically, Gottman and Katz (1989) found indirect paths indicating that parents in distressed marriages who are physiologically underaroused have a cold, unresponsive, inadequately structured parenting style, which relates to anger and noncompliance in children and high levels of stress-related hormones. These children's peer play is characterized by less play and more negativity, and these children are not as healthy as children from homes with parents in nondistressed marriages. Other direct paths indicated that children whose parents' marriage is discordant are under chronic stress, as demonstrated by high levels of urinary catecholamines. A second study by Gottman and colleagues (Hooven, Gottman, & Katz, 1995) also links parents' behavior to children's health. In a longitudinal study of marriage, parents were interviewed when their children were preschoolers, and again when their children were 8 years old, about their marriages. Observations were also made of how well parents helped their children manage frustration and anger in two laboratory contexts. Parents who understood and accepted their own emotions, as measured by how they described their marriages, and who actively helped their children to think about their emotions and express them in acceptable ways, had children with lower levels of stress hormones in their urine and a lower heart rate. Viewed together, these studies suggest that experiencing parental marital anger and other negative emotions can be very stressful for children, resulting in distress, arousal, and eventually compromised physical health. Moreover, these patterns of childhood reactivity to parental emotions may contribute to aggressive response patterns to others (Cummings, 1998). For example, research by Dodge and his associates (Crick & Dodge, 1996; Dodge, 1985) suggests that children who view hostility at home may come to perceive hostile intent in otherwise ambiguous situations and respond in an inappropriately aggressive manner. Responding in this manner to ambiguous situations may then cause others to react aggressively and result in more frequent conflicts in many contexts outside the family, further contributing to children's health risk. However, other parental behaviors may buffer children's health risk associated with marital discord. Other studies have found that maternal support can temper the health impact of stressful life events in childhood. Furthermore, although it appears that stressful parental interactions with others may be physiologically harmful to children, recent evidence provided by Katz and Gottman (1994) suggests an intriguing alternative hypothesis. This research demonstrated that in intact marriages, it is better for children if the parents engage in conflict when resolving marital differences than if they withdraw from each other. When parents withdraw from each other, children increase their expressions of anger and physiological responses indicating an inability to regulate affect. These researchers stated that perhaps conflictive marital interaction is perceived by children as active problem solving, especially if the children are privy to the resolution (Cummings, Vogel, Cummings, & El-Sheikh, 1989). Perhaps parents in marriages characterized by withdrawal are signaling to the children that the relationship is about to end. This message is more stressful and causes greater negative physiological response than the message delivered by a mother who is angry with her spouse yet engaged in the relationship (Katz & Gottman, 1994).

The mechanisms by which children's negative emotional states, as influenced by parents' marital discord, result in compromised physical health are not established. From a direct-effects perspective, parents' negative emotional states could result in inadequate attention to children's health behavior and needs. For example, maternal depression (Downey & Coyne, 1990) was implicated in a variety of maladaptive parenting behaviors. From a health perspective, maternal negative emotional states, such as depression, could result in infrequent use of wellness services for children (e.g., immunizations, well-child exams) and inadequate monitoring of children's daily preventive health behavior.

Indirect effects of parents' negative emotional states on children's health behavior can also be delineated. A mother's anger or hostility toward her physician or the health system in general could lead her to ignore important symptoms, which in turn could result in her morbidity or mortality – a significant stressor in childhood. Thus, a variety of direct and indirect effects of parents' negative emotional states can influence children's health behavior and status.

These studies suggest that research exploring the relations between children's emotional climate, of which the parents are prime architects, and health is maturing and is being examined as a more fully contextualized issue. One factor influencing children's emotional climate, and consequentially their health, which I have not yet discussed, is the multiple roles of parents. Although some research has suggested that the juggling of roles in which modern parents engage is deleterious to their health, some recent research suggests that employment, marriage, and parenthood are actually associated with good physical health for both men and women (Verbrugge, 1983). Employed married parents tend to have the best health profiles, while persons with none of these roles have the worst health profiles. In fact, men and women with both job and family roles enjoy the health benefits of each role and incur no special health disadvantage in fulfilling both roles. Whether these findings are accounted for by reduced health risks for socially active people, less sensitivity to symptoms exhibited by busy persons, or social selection in which healthy people are able to acquire and maintain roles more easily than unhealthy people is unclear. It is encouraging to know that parenthood per se does not negatively affect parents' health; nevertheless, parents often become acutely and chronically ill. In light of these findings, I now turn to an examination of the impact of parents' health on children's health.

The Impact of Parents' Health on Children's Health

A relatively new area of research concerns the effect of parents' health status on children's health. All parents experience minor acute illnesses periodically while rearing their children, and more than 10 million adults under the age of 45 years suffer limitation of activity associated with chronic illness (Benson & Marano, 1998). Most researchers who study familial socialization of childhood health behavior and outcomes ignore this aspect of how parents influence their children's health (Drotar, 1994). However, investigators are becoming increasingly aware of how such parental health behavior as cigarette smoking impacts both childhood behavior (e.g., childhood cigarette smoking, as discussed earlier) and childhood health (e.g., the deleterious effects of secondhand smoke) (Leftwich & Collins, 1994). In fact, recent evidence suggests striking effects of mothers' smoking during pregnancy on daughters' smoking behavior. Kandel and her colleagues (Kandel, Wu, & Davies, 1994) found that mothers' smoking during pregnancy increased the probability that daughters would smoke and continue to smoke during adolescence. These researchers hypothesize that nicotine or other associated substances from cigarettes predispose fetal nervous systems to addictive behavior later in life.

Other maternal health problems that are known to affect children through biological channels are maternal crack and cocaine use and HIV infection (Black, Nair, & Harrington, 1994; Drotar, 1994; Singer, Arendt, Farkas, & Minnes, 1997). In an elegant analysis of the conceptual and methodological concerns inherent in defining the effect of parental health problems on children, Drotar (1994) has outlined several important considerations. These include the nature and duration of children's exposure to parents' health problems, the pathways and mechanisms through which parents' health problems impact on children, and individual differences in the influence of parents' health problems on children (e.g., developmental, risk, and resiliency factors).

In a comprehensive study of the effect of parental physical symptoms and health services utilization on children, Stein and Newcomb (1994) found that maternal reporting of a greater number of major health problems in the past 4 years predicted more psychosomatic complaints in their children. Although the cross-sectional nature of this study does not permit questions of causality to be answered, these results suggest either a social learning or biological predisposition explanation. Another study tested a similar hypothesis: that the prior experience of physical illness in childhood is associated with later experience of medically unexplained symptoms (Hotopf, Mayou, Wadsworth, & Wessely, 1999). The 5% of most symptomatic individuals at age 36 years participating in a large prospective birth cohort study were identified and screened for physical illness. Subjects without defined physical diagnoses were compared with the remainder of the sample for childhood exposure to family medical illness. A powerful relation was demonstrated between poor reported health of parents when the subjects were 15 years of age and their own symptoms at age 36, independent of their current psychiatric status. The authors of this study conclude that medically unexplained symptoms in adulthood appear to be related to childhood experience of family illness, and may reflect a learned process whereby illness experience leads to symptom monitoring. Regardless, these data indicate the salience of parents' health status and behavior for children's health behavior (Garralda, 2000).

Parmelee (1986, 1997) has argued for examining the specific ways in which parents socialize their children concerning how to respond to recurring minor illness. As children become ill with minor contagious acute illnesses and share them with their parents, Parmelee suggests that children are provided with repetitive opportunities to observe and participate in the care of their father or mother who is experiencing what they have experienced. Parmelee believes that this helps children develop an understanding of the feelings of others, and that these shared personal illness experiences are an important beneficial aspect of children's social growth experience, in addition to providing models of sick role behavior. Very young children are quite capable of empathic behavior (Zahn-Waxler, Radke-Yarrow, & King, 1979), and in combination with the salience of physical symptoms for young children (Bretherton & Beeghly, 1982), parents' minor illnesses provide a potent learning resource for childhood socialization (Parmelee, 1986).

Others cite the opportunity for further elaboration of children's sex role attitudes in parents' illness. For example, when a mother is ill, the father must often take over some of her duties, such as preparing meals or doing laundry (Wilkinson, 1988). In addition to observing behavior of the caretaking parent that violates stereotyped family role behaviors, these events offer children role models of how to respond as a male or female to family illness (Wilkinson, 1988).

As Wilkinson (1988) suggests, "Illness represents a challenge to established practices which we develop for living together; it makes demands on our role flexibility and sensitivity to each other. Children have their own impressions of these effects. . . . " (p. 85).

Finally, family rituals during illness that are established in childhood may provide comfort and stability throughout life. Because illness can threaten the security of normal attachment relationships, the socially approved illness roles that children observe and learn in the context of family members' illness may provide a stabilizing influence during the periods of uncertainty that characterize acute and chronic illness (Douglas, 1966; Wilkinson, 1988; Wolin & Bennett, 1984).

9

Summary and Conclusions

Throughout this book, I have reviewed the results of many studies of how children learn to be healthy. I have described and critiqued a variety of theories that attempt to explain and interpret the detailed and highly complex information compiled by theorists and researchers in their effort to understand children's health learning and behavior. Neither data nor the many theories advanced are final answers in the continuing attempt to unravel the puzzles of children's health. As in any field of science, our information about how children learn to be healthy is constantly expanding and changing.

Research on influences on children's health attitudes and behaviors has now achieved considerable momentum, accompanied by an increase in attempts to model these multiple influences, as indicated throughout this book. In this final chapter, I wish to reiterate some of the broad themes that I have emphasized in the preceding chapters concerning how children learn to be healthy. First, these compiled theories and studies illustrate that children experience both continuity and discontinuity in the health information they receive from socialization agents such as the family, peers, schools, and the media. Thus, the burden of integrating health socialization falls on the child. However, when these agents of socialization are coordinated in their efforts to modify children's health attitudes and behavior, success rates are often higher. Even media usage can be coordinated to provide consistency across the socialization offered by parents, schools, and peers.

Second, children's knowledge and understanding of health progresses in a developmental fashion, with greater quantity, sophistication, and complexity of understanding of health being apparent in older versus younger children. Although some evidence suggests that the development of children's health knowledge is similar to the emergence of children's understanding in other areas (e.g., moral development), more work is needed to determine the extent to which understanding of health is domain specific or follows a developmental progression shared with other areas of children's knowledge.

Third, an individual differences perspective promises to improve the power of our explanatory models of children's health attitudes and behavior. Models that combine information on psychosocial dimensions (e.g., self-esteem, locus of control) with influences of socialization agents (e.g., the mother's attitudes toward health behavior, parents' intelligence) are able to explain substantial amounts of variance in children's health attitudes and behavior.

The current models are limited for a number of reasons, including their reliance on self-report and cross-sectional data. Each of these models tends to focus on only a few of the influences that have been demonstrated, in this book, to affect children's health attitudes and behavior. With the accumulation of studies documenting the multiple influences involved in the socialization of children's health attitudes and behavior, the requirements for a meaningful model of children's health attitudes and behavior have become more complex. This book has identified additional important sets of domains that must also be considered in efforts to understand the development of children's health attitudes and behavior, including demographic variables, psychosocial dimensions, and the influence of various socialization agents. No one study can be expected to address all of these, but cognizant of this complexity, researchers should be cautious in interpreting the results of studies that do not address the multiple sources of influence in children's health socialization.

Fourth, greater attention must be given to specifying the developmental changes in socialization of children's health attitudes and behavior. As in other domains of development, the strength of influence of cognitive development, psychological health, and socialization agents ebbs and flows over the course of children's health development, and models that emphasize various aspects of these influences, depending on the child's developmental status, will have to be developed.

Fifth, the direction-of-effects issue permeates the area of children's physical health. Many variables affecting children's health attitudes and behavior appear to be affected by children's health attitudes as well. For example, as noted earlier in this book, self-esteem appears to be influenced by children's perception of wellness and their knowledge about health processes, but also is found to influence children's health attitudes and expectations about health behavior (Bush & Iannotti, 1990). Greater attention to the specification of direction of effects in future models of child health attitudes and behavior is suggested by such data.

Sixth, the pathways of influence, regardless of direction, may not always be direct. Instead, the relation variables in models of child health attitudes and behavior may be mediated by additional variables (Lau & Klepper, 1988). Again, these possibilities must be evident in our models of these processes. This is nicely illustrated by Bush and Iannotti (1990); socioeconomic status has significant indirect effects along many paths.

Seventh, more attention needs to be paid to the influence of ethnicity, gender, and socioeconomic status on the processes associated with children's health socialization. Although traditional views of children's health have utilized demographic variables in attempts to describe and predict the impact of families on children's health status, few studies have examined the effects of these factors on the family socialization process and dynamics with respect to children's acquisition of health attitudes and behaviors.

Eighth, interview and survey studies have dominated the research on children's health learning and behavior, to the almost complete exclusion of studies utilizing observational methods. Process-oriented observational studies of how families make decisions concerning their children's health issues (i.e., family child health risk management), parent–child health-related interactions, and peer influence on children's health attitudes and behavior are necessary to further inform us about the mechanisms of children's health socialization and learning. Moreover, studies of children's health attitudes utilizing nonfamilial informants (e.g., peers, teachers, pediatricians) are important, and currently are mostly neglected sources of data on children's health attitudes and behavior.

Ninth, the mechanisms of children's health-related attitude and behavior acquisition and socialization deserve more attention at both the theoretical and empirical levels. Two issues merit exploration. First, what familial or other social environmental conditions provide the opportunity to acquire attitudes or behaviors that are necessary for wellness? Second, what are the mechanisms that facilitate the acquisition and socialization of these attitudes and behaviors?

The research to date has focused on several possible factors that may be involved in explaining childhood health socialization. In studies of children's health attitudes and behavior, the explanatory burden has fallen on three categories of variables: (1) children's background and characteristics (i.e., developmental status, demographics, personality variables, and possibly gender), (2) parents' and families' relational and interaction variables, and (3) extrafamilial agents (peers, schools, media).

The most common and well-researched way in which children learn about health is through familial relationships. Research documents that parents and families provide models of health attitudes and behavior, demonstrating, teaching, and reinforcing specific health attitudes and behavior, as influenced by background characteristics such as demographics and parents' personality variables. Children are hypothesized to learn concepts of health and health skills by being given repeated opportunities to practice these behaviors at home. Evidence suggests that these concepts and skills are utilized by children, as they get older, in other health behavior–eliciting situations, such as with peers and in school. Exposure to these alternate contexts serves to modify these health attitudes and behaviors, but nevertheless, the research indicates that children's health attitudes and behaviors appear to be more similar than dissimilar to those of their parents.

Future studies of the acquisition and socialization of children's health attitudes and behavior should involve both the specification of important individual variables and the testing of overarching models. The etiology of children's health attitudes and behavior warrants more sustained and systematic inquiry in our quest for helping children to be as healthy as they can be.

References

Adams, G. R., Hicken, M., & Salehi, M. (1988). Socialization of the physical attractiveness stereotype: Parental expectations and verbal behaviors. *International Journal of Psychology, 23*, 137–149.

Adler, N. E., Boyce, T., Chesney, M. A., Cohen, S., Folkman, S., Kahn, D., & Syme, S. (1994). Socioeconomic status and health: The challenge of the gradient. *American Psychologist, 49*, 15–24.

Affleck, G., McGrade, B. J., Allen, D. A., & McQueeney, M. (1985). Mothers' beliefs about behavioral causes for their developmentally disabled infant's condition: What do they signify? *Journal of Pediatric Psychology, 10*, 293–303.

Ainsworth, M. D., Blehar, M., Waters, E., & Wall, S. (1978). *Patterns of attachment*. Hillsdale, NJ: Erlbaum.

Almarsdottir, A. B., & Zimmer, C. (1998). Children's knowledge about medicines. *Childhood: A Global Journal of Child Research, 5*, 265–281.

American Academy of Pediatrics. (2000a). Race/ethnicity, gender, socioeconomic status-research exploring their effects on child health: A subject review. *Pediatrics, 105*, 1349–1351.

(2000b). School health assessments. *Pediatrics, 105*, 875–877.

American Health Foundation. (1995). *First national child health survey*. New York: American Health Foundation.

Andersen, R. E., Crespo, C. J., Bartlett, S. J., Cheskin, L. J., & Pratt, M. (1998). Relationship of physical activity and television watching with body weight and level of fatness among children. *Journal of the American Medical Association, 279*, 938–942.

Anderson, D. R., Huston, A. C., Schmitt, K. L., Linebarger, D. L., & Wright, J. C. (2001). Early childhood television viewing and adolescent behavior. *Monographs of the Society for Research in Child Development, 65.*

Armstrong, C. A., Sallis, J. F., Alcaraz, J. E., Kolody, B., McKenzie, T. L., & Hovell, M. F. (1998). Children's television viewing, body fat, and physical fitness. *American Journal of Health Promotion, 12,* 363–368.

Asher, S. R., Rose, A. J., & Gabriel, S. W. (2001). Peer rejection in everyday life. In M. R. Leary (Ed.), *Interpersonal rejection* (pp. 105–142). New York: Oxford University Press.

Atkin, C. K. (1990). Effects of televised alcohol messages on teenage drinking patterns. *Journal of Adolescent Health Care, 11,* 10–24.

Au, T. K., Romo, L. F., & DeWitt, J. E. (1999). Considering children's folkbiology in health education. In M. Siegal & C. C. Petersen (Eds.), *Children's understanding of biology and health* (pp. 209–234). New York: Cambridge University Press.

Auslander, W. F., Haire-Joshu, D., Rogge, M., & Santiago, J. V. (1991). Predictors of diabetes knowledge in newly diagnosed children and parents. *Journal of Pediatric Psychology, 16,* 213–228.

Austin, E. W., & Johnson, K. (1997). Effects of general and alcohol-specific media literacy training on children's decision making about alcohol. *Journal of Health Communication, 2,* 17–42.

Aylward, G. P. (1992). The relationship between environmental risk and developmental outcome. *Journal of Developmental and Behavioral Pediatrics, 13,* 222–229.

Bacon, M. K., & Ashmore, R. D. (1985). How mothers and fathers categorize descriptions of social behavior attributed to daughters and sons. *Social Cognition, 3,* 193–217.

Baeyer, C. L., & Walker, L. S. (1999). Children with recurrent abdominal pain: Issues in the selection and description of research participants. *Journal of Developmental and Behavioral Pediatrics, 20,* 307–313.

Baker-Ward, L., Gordon, B. N., Ornstein, P. A., Larus, D. M., & Clubb, P. A. (1993). Young children's long-term retention of a pediatric examination. *Child Development, 64,* 1519–1533.

Baldwin, A. L., Baldwin, C., & Cole, R. E. (1990). Stress-resistant families and stress-resistant children. In J. E. Rolf & A. S. Masten (Eds.), *Risk and protective factors in the development of psychopathology* (pp. 257–280). New York: Cambridge University Press.

Baldwin, S. E., & Baranowski, M. V. (1990). Family interactions and sex education in the home. *Adolescence, 25,* 573–582.

Bandura, A. (1989). Cognitive social learning theory. In R. Vasta (Ed.), *Annals of child development,* Vol. 6: *Six theories of child development: Revised formulations and current issues* (pp. 1–60). Greenwich, CT: JAI Press.

Barcus, F. E. (1987). *Food advertising on children's television: An analysis of appeals and nutritional content.* Newtonville, MA: Action for Children's Television.

Bartlett, E. E. (1981). The contribution of school health education to community health promotion: What can we reasonably expect? *American Journal of Public Health, 71,* 1384–1391.

Bauchner, H., McCarthy, P. L., Sznajderman, S. D., & Baron, M. A. (1987). Do mothers overestimate the seriousness of their infants' acute illnesses? *Journal of Developmental & Behavioral Pediatrics, 8,* 255–259.

Bauchner, H., Waring, C., & Vinci, R. (1991). Parental presence during procedures in an emergency room: Results from 50 observations. *Pediatrics, 87,* 544–548.

Bauman, K. E., Ennett, S. T., Foshee, V. A., & Pemberton, M. (2001). Correlates of participation in a family-directed tobacco and alcohol prevention program for adolescents. *Health Education & Behavior, 28,* 440–461.

Baumeister, L. M., Flores, E., & Marin, B. V. (1995). Sex information given to Latina adolescents by parents. *Health Education Research, 10,* 233–239.

Baumrind, D. (1978). Parental disciplinary patterns and social competence in youth. *Youth and Society, 9,* 239–278.

Becker, M. H., & Green, L. W. (1975). A family approach to compliance with medical treatment: A selective review of the literature. *International Journal of Health Education, 18,* 173–182.

Becker, M. H., Maiman, L., Kirscht, J., Haefner, D., & Drachman, R. (1977). The health belief model and dietary compliance: A field experiment. *Journal of Health and Social Behavior, 18,* 348–366.

Bejerot, N. (1980). Addiction to pleasure: A biological and social-psychological theory of addiction. In D. J. Lettieri, M. Sayers, & H. W. Pearson (Eds.), *Theories on drug abuse: Selected contemporary perspectives* (NIDA Research Monograph 30) (pp. 114–132). Rockville, MD: National Institute on Drug Abuse.

Bennett, S. M., Huntsman, E., & Lilley, C. M. (2000). Parent perceptions of the impact of chronic pain in children and adolescents. *Children's Health Care, 29,* 147–159.

Benson, V., & Marano, M. A. (1998). Current estimates from the National Health Interview Survey, 1995. *Vital and Health Statistics. Series 10: Data from the National Health Survey, 199,* 1–428.

Berger, D. M. (1980). *The relationship between health locus of control and health values of the mother and immunization levels of her children.* Unpublished master's thesis, Virginia Commonwealth University, Richmond.

Bernard, P. A., Johnston, C., Curtis, S. E., & King, W. D. (1998). Toppled television sets cause significant pediatric morbidity and mortality. *Pediatrics, 102*, 32.

Berndt, T. J. (1989). Obtaining social support from friends in childhood and adolescence. In D. Belle (Ed.), *Children's social networks and social supports* (pp. 308–331). New York: Wiley.

Berne, L. A., Patton, W., Milton, J., & Hunt, L. Y. A. (2000). A qualitative assessment of Australian parents' perceptions of sexuality education and communication. *Journal of Sex Education and Therapy, 25*, 161–168.

Bibace, R., & Walsh, M. W. (1980). Development of children's concepts of illness. *Pediatrics, 66*, 912–917.

Birch, L. L., Marlin, D. W., & Rotter, J. (1984). Eating as the "means" activity in a contingency: Effects on young children's food preference. *Child Development, 55*, 431–439.

Black, M. M., Nair, P., & Harrington, D. (1994). Maternal HIV infection: Parenting and early child development. *Journal of Pediatric Psychology, 19*, 595–615.

Blum, R. W. (2001). Trends in adolescent health: Perspectives from the United States. *International Journal of Adolescent Medicine and Health, 13*, 287–295.

Blum, R. W., Beuhring, T., Shew, M. L., & Bearinger, L. H. (2000). The effects of race/ethnicity, income, and family structure on adolescent risk behaviors. *American Journal of Public Health, 90*, 1879–1884.

Borzekowski, D. L. G. (1996). Embedded anti-alcohol messages on commercial television: What teenagers perceive. *Journal of Adolescent Health, 19*, 345–352.

Borzekowski, D. L. G., Robinson, T. N., & Killen, J. D. (2000). Does the camera add 10 pounds? Media use, perceived importance of appearance, and weight concerns among teenage girls. *Journal of Adolescent Health, 26*, 36–41.

Bowser, B. P., & Wingood, G. M. (1992). Community-based HIV-prevention programs for adolescents. In E. R. J. DiClemente (Ed.), *Adolescents and HIV: A generation in jeopardy* (pp. 194–211). Newbury Park, CA: Sage.

Bretherton, I., & Beeghly, M. (1982). Talking about internal states: The acquisition of an explicit theory of mind. *Developmental Psychology, 18*, 906–921.

Brock, L. J., & Jennings, G. H. (1993). What daughters in their 30s wish their mothers had told them. *Family Relations, 42*, 61–65.

Brody, G. H., Flor, D., Hollett-Wright, N., McCoy, J. K., & Donovan, J. (1999). Parent–child relationships, child temperament profiles, and children's alcohol use norms. *Journal of Studies on Alcohol, Supplement 13*, 45–51.

Bronfenbrenner, U. (2000). Environments in developmental perspective: Theoretical and operational models. In S. L. Friedman & T. E. Wachs (Eds.), *Measuring environment across the life span: Emerging methods and concepts* (pp. 3–28). Washington, DC: American Psychological Association.

Brooks-Gunn, J., Duncan, G. J., Klebanov, P. K., & Sealand, N. (1993). Do neighborhoods influence child and adolescent development? *American Journal of Sociology*, *99*, 353–395.

Broome, M. E., & Endsley, R. (1989). Parent and child behavior during immunization. *Pain*, *37*, 85–92.

Broome, M. E., Richtsmeier, A., Maikler, V., & Alexander, M. (1986). Pediatric pain practices: A national survey of health professionals. *Journal of Pain and Symptom Management*, *11*, 312–320.

Brown, B. B. (1990). Peer groups and peer cultures. In S. S. Feldman & B. R. Elliot (Eds.), *At the threshold: The developing adolescent.* Washington, DC: Carnegie Corporation.

Brown, J. D. (2000). Adolescents' sexual media diets. *Journal of Adolescent Health*, *27*, 35–40.

Brown, J. D., Childers, K. W., & Waszak, C. S. (1990). Television and adolescent sexuality. *Journal of Adolescent Health Care*, *11*, 62–70.

Brown, J. D., & Hayes, T. (2001). Family attitudes towards television. In J. Bryant & J. A. Bryant (Eds.), *Television and the American family* (pp. 111–138). Mahwah, NJ: Erlbaum.

Brown, J D., & Newcomer, S. F. (1991). Influences of television and peers on adolescents' sexual behavior. *Journal of Homosexuality*, *21*, 77–91.

Broyles, S. L., Nader, P. R., Sallis, J. F., & Frank-Spohrer, G. C. (1996). Cardiovascular disease risk factors in Anglo and Mexican American children and their mothers. *Family and Community Health*, *19*, 57–72.

Bruck, M., Ceci, S. J., Francoeur, E., & Barr, R. (1995). "I hardly cried when I got my shot!": Influencing children's reports about a visit to their pediatrician. *Child Development*, *66*, 193–208.

Bruhn, J. G., & Cordova, F. D. (1977). A developmental approach to learning wellness behavior: Infancy to early adolescence. *Health Values*, *1*, 246–254.

Bryant, J., & Bryant, J. A. (Eds.). (2001). *Television and the American family*. Mahwah, NJ: Erlbaum.

Burbach, D. J., & Peterson, L. (1986). Children's concepts of physical illness: A review and critique of the cognitive-developmental literature. *Health Psychology*, *5*, 307–325.

Bush, J. P., & Iannotti, R. J. (1988). Origins and stability of children's health beliefs relative to medicine use. *Social Science and Medicine*, *27*, 315–352.

Bush, J. P., & Iannotti, R. J. (1990). A children's health belief model. *Medical Care*, *28*, 69–80.

Bush, J. P., Melamed, B. G., Sheras, P. L., & Greenbaum, P. E. (1986). Mother–child patterns of coping with anticipatory medical stress. *Health Psychology*, *5*, 137–157.

Bush, J. P., Young, S. R., & Radecki-Bush, C. (1998). The child as a collaborator in pediatric pain management: Implications for clinical practice. *Psychotherapy in Private Practice*, *17*, 43–61.

Butler, J. A., Starfield, B., & Stenmark, S. (1984). Child health policy. In H. W. Stevenson & A. E. Siegel (Eds.), *Child development research and social policy* (pp. 110–179). Chicago: University of Chicago Press.

Byrd-Bredbenner, C., & Grasso, D. (2000). Health, medicine, and food messages in television commercials during 1992 and 1998. *Journal of School Health*, *70*, 61–65.

Cairns, R. B., & Cairns, B. D. (1994). *Lifelines and risks: Pathways of youth in our time*. New York: Cambridge University Press.

Campbell, J. D. (1975). Illness is a point of view: The development of children's concepts of illness. *Child Development*, *46*, 92–100.

   (1978). Studies in attitude formation: Development of health orientations. In C. W. Sherif & M. Sherif (Eds.), *Attitude, ego-involvement and change* (pp. 35–51). New York: Wiley.

Campion, P. D., & Gabriel, J. (1985). Illness behaviour in mothers with young children. *Social Science and Medicine*, *20*, 325–330.

Carey, S. (1985). *Conceptual change in childhood*. London: Methuen.

Carlson, C. I., Tharinger, D. J., Bricklin, P. M., & DeMers, S. T. (1996). Health care reform and psychological practice in schools. *Professional Psychology: Research and Practice*, *27*, 14–23.

Carlson, L., Laczniak, R. N., & Walsh, A. (2001). Socializing children about television: An intergenerational study. *Journal of the Academy of Marketing Science*, *29*, 276–288.

Carpenter, E. S. (1990). Children's health care and the changing role of women. *Medical Care*, *18*, 1208–1218.

Centers for Disease Control and Prevention. (1991). Effectiveness in disease and injury prevention characteristics of parents who discuss AIDS with their children – United States, 1989. *Morbidity and Mortality Weekly Report*, *40*, 789–791.

Charren, P. (1985). Children's television: A national disgrace. *Pediatrics Annual*, *14*, 822–827.

Children's Defense Fund. (1988). *A call for action to make our nation safe for children: A briefing book on the status of American children in 1988*. Washington, DC: Author.

Children's Defense Fund. (1994). *The state of America's children yearbook, 1994*. New York: Author.

Christ, M. J., Raszkat, W. V., & Dillon, C. A. (1998). Prioritizing education about condom use among sexually active female adolescents.
Adolescence, 33, 735–744.

Christoffel, K. K., & Christoffel, T. (1986). Handguns as a pediatric
problem. *Pediatric Emergency Care, 2,* 75–81.

Christopherson, C. R., Miller, B. C., & Norton, M. C. (1994, April).
*Pubertal development, parent–teen communication, and sexual values
as predictors of adolescent sexual intentions and sexually related behaviors.* Paper presented at the meeting of the Society for Research
on Adolescence, San Diego.

Clarke-Stewart, A. (1993). *Daycare.* Cambridge, MA: Harvard University
Press.

Cohen, L. L., Manimala, R., & Blount, R. L. (2000). Easier said than
done: What parents say they do and what they do during children's
immunizations. *Children's Health Care, 29,* 79–86.

Coie, J. D., & Dodge, K. A. (1998). Aggression and antisocial behavior.
In W. Damon (Gen. Ed.) and N. Eisenberg (Vol. Ed.), *Handbook of
child psychology,* Vol. 3: *Social, emotional, and personality development* (pp. 779–862). New York: Wiley.

Compas, B. E., Connor-Smith, J. K., Saltzman, H., & Thomsen, A. H.
(2001). Coping with stress during childhood and adolescence: Problems, progress, and potential in theory and research. *Psychological
Bulletin, 127,* 87–127.

Compas, B. E., & Harding Thomsen, A. (1999). Coping and responses
to stress among children with recurrent abdominal pain. *Journal of
Developmental and Behavioral Pediatrics, 20,* 323–324.

Comstock, G., & Paik, H. (1991). *Television and the American child.*
New York: Academic Press.

Cooper, P. F., & Weinick, R. M. (1999). The impact of fathers on children's
health care. *Abstract Book: Association for Health Services Research,
16,* 142–143.

Coulton, C. L., & Pandey, S. (1992). Geographic concentration of poverty
and risk to children in urban neighborhoods. *American Behavioral
Scientist, 35,* 238–257.

Coyne-Beasley, T., & Schoenbach, V. J. (2000). The African-American
church: A potential forum for adolescent comprehensive sexuality
education. *Journal of Adolescent Health, 26,* 289–294.

Crawford, I., Jason, L. A., Riordan, N., & Kaufman, J. (1990). A
multimedia-based approach to increasing communication and the
level of HIV knowledge within families. Special issue: HIV and the
community. *Journal of Community Psychology, 18,* 361–373.

Crawford, I., Thomas, S., & Zoller, D. (1993). Communication and level
of HIV knowledge among homeless African-American mothers and
their children. *Journal of Health and Social Policy, 4,* 37–53.

Crick, N., & Dodge, K. (1994). A review and reformulation of social information-processing mechanisms in children's social adjustment. *Psychological Bulletin, 115*, 74–101.

(1996). Social information-processing mechanisms on reactive and proactive aggression. *Child Development, 67*, 993–1002.

Crider, C. (1981). Children's conceptions of the body interior. In R. Bibace & M. Walsh (Eds.), *New directions for child development: Children's conceptions of health, illness, and bodily functions*, No. 14. San Francisco: Jossey-Bass.

Croft, C. A., & Asmussen, L. (1992). Perceptions of mothers, youth, and educators: A path toward detente regarding sexuality education. *Family Relations, 41*, 452–459.

Crooks, D. L. (2000). Food consumption, activity, and overweight among school children in an Appalachian Kentucky community. *American Journal of Physical Anthropology, 112*, 159–170.

Crosby, R. A., DiClemente, R. J., Wingood, G. M., Sionean, C., Cobb, B. K., & Harrington, K. (2000). Correlates of unprotected vaginal sex among African American female adolescents. *Archives of Adolescent Medicine, 154*, 893–899.

Cummings, E. M. (1998). Stress and coping approaches and research: The impact of marital conflict on children. *Journal of Aggression, Maltreatment and Trauma, 2*, 31–50.

Cummings, E. M., Goeke-Morey, M. C., & Dukewich, T. L. (2001). The study of relations between marital conflict and child adjustment: Challenges and new directions for methodology. In J. H. Grych & F. D. Fincham (Eds.), *Interparental conflict and child development: Theory, research, and applications* (pp. 39–63). New York: Cambridge University Press.

Cummings, E. M., Vogel, D., Cummings, J. S., & El-Sheikh, M. (1989). Children's response to different forms of expression of anger between adults. *Child Development, 60*, 1392–1404.

Dallas, C., Wilson, T., & Salgado, V. (2000). Gender differences in teen parents' perceptions of parental responsibilities. *Public Health Nursing, 17*, 423–433.

Darling, C. A., & Hicks, M. W. (1982). Parental influence on adolescent sexuality: Implications for parents as educators. *Journal of Youth and Adolescence, 11*, 231–245.

Davis, C., Noel, M. B., Chan, S.-F., & Wing, L. S. (1998). Knowledge, attitudes, and behaviours related to HIV and HIV among Chinese adolescents in Hong Kong. *Journal of Adolescence, 21*, 657–665.

Davison, K. K., & Birch, L. L. (2001). Weight status, parent reaction, and self-concept in five-year-old girls. *Pediatrics, 107*, 46–53.

de Foe, J. R., & Breed, W. (1988). Youth and alcohol in television stories, with suggestions to the industry for alternative portrayals. *Adolescence, 23,* 533–550.

DeJong, W., & Hoffman, K. D. (2000). A content analysis of television advertising for the Massachusetts Tobacco Control Media Campaign, 1993–1996. *Journal of Public Health Management and Practice, 6,* 27–39.

DeMers, S. T., & Bricklin, P. (1995). Legal, professional, and financial constraints on psychologists' delivery of health care services in school settings. *School Psychology Quarterly, 10,* 217–235.

DeVellis, R. F., DeVellis, B. M., Revicki, D. M., Lurie, S. F., Runyan, C. W., & Bristol, M. (1986). Development and validation of the Child Improvement Locus of Control (CILC) Scales. *Journal of Social and Clinical Psychology, 3,* 307–324.

Diaz, R. M., Neal, C. J., & Vachio, A. (1991). Maternal teaching in the zone of proximal development: A comparison of low- and high-risk dyads. *Merrill-Palmer Quarterly, 37,* 83–107.

Dielman, T. E., Leech, S. L., Becker, M. H., Rosenstock, I. R., Horvath, B. F., & Radius, S. M. (1982). Parental and child health beliefs and behavior. *Health Education Quarterly, 9,* 156–173.

Die-Trill, M., Bromberg, J., LaVally, B., & Portales, L. A. (1996). Development of social skills in boys with brain tumors: A group approach. *Journal of Psychosocial Oncology, 14,* 23–41.

Dietz, W. H., & Gortmaker, S. L. (1985). Do we fatten our children at the television set? Obesity and television viewing in children and adolescents. *Pediatrics, 75,* 807–812.

DiIorio, C., Kelley, M., & Hockenberry-Eaton, M. (1999). Communication about sexual issues: Mothers, fathers, and friends. *Journal of Adolescent Health, 24,* 181–189.

DiIorio, C., Resnicow, K., Dudley, W. N., Thomas, S., Wang, D. T., Van Marter, D. F., Manteuffel, B., & Lipana, J. (2000). Social cognitive factors associated with mother–adolescent communication. *Journal of Health Communication, 5,* 41–51.

DiLiberti, J. H. (2000). The relationship between social stratification and all-cause mortality. *Pediatrics, 105,* 35–47.

Dix, T., & Grusec, J. E. (1983). Parental influence techniques: An attributional analysis. *Child Development, 54,* 645–652.

Dix, T., & Reinhold, D. P. (1991). Chronic and temporary influences on mothers' attributions for children's disobedience. *Merrill-Palmer Quarterly, 37,* 251–271.

Dodge, K. A. (1985). A social information processing model of social competence in children. In M. Perlmutter (Ed.), *Minnesota Symposium on Child Psychology* (Vol. 18, pp. 77–126). Hillsdale, NJ: Erlbaum.

Dodge, K. A. (1991). Emotion and social information processing. In J. Garber & K. A. Dodge (Eds.), *The development of emotion regulation and dysregulation* (pp. 159–181). New York: Cambridge University Press.

Dodge, K. A., & Somberg, D. R. (1987). Hostile attributional biases among aggressive boys are exacerbated under conditions of threats to the self. *Child Development, 58*, 213–224.

Doherty, W. J., & Allen, W. (1994). Family functioning and parental smoking as predictors of adolescent cigarette use: A six-year prospective study. *Journal of Family Psychology, 8*, 347–353.

Doherty, W. J., & Campbell, T. L. (1988). *Families and health*. Newbury Park, CA: Sage.

Donovan, J. E., Jessor, R., & Costa, F. M. (1991). Adolescent health behavior and conventionality-unconventionality: An extension of problem-behavior therapy. *Health Psychology, 10*, 52–61.

Dorr, A., Kovaric, P., & Doubleday, C. (1989). Parent–child coviewing of television. *Journal of Broadcasting and Electronic Media, 33*, 35–51.

Douglas, M. (1966). *Purity and danger: An analysis of concepts of pollution and taboo*. London: Routledge and Kegan Paul.

Dowden, S. L., Calvert, R. D., Davis, L., & Gullotta, T. P. (1997). Improving access to health care: School-based health centers. In R. P. Weissberg & T. P. Gullotta (Eds.), *Healthy children 2010: Establishing preventive services* (pp. 154–182). Thousand Oaks, CA: Sage.

Downey, G., & Coyne, J. C. (1990). Children of depressed parents: An integrative review. *Psychological Bulletin, 108*, 50–76.

Drotar, D. (1981). Psychological perspectives in chronic childhood illness. *Journal of Pediatric Psychology, 6*, 211–228.

Drotar, D. (1994). Impact of parental health problems on children: Concepts, methods, and unanswered questions. *Journal of Pediatric Psychology, 19*, 525–536.

Drotar, D., & Robinson, J. (2000). Developmental psychopathology of failure to thrive. In A. J. Sameroff & M. Lewis (Eds.), *Handbook of developmental psychopathology* (2nd ed., pp. 351–364). New York: Kluwer.

Dryfoos, J. G. (1994). *Full-service schools: A revolution in health and social services for children, youth, and families*. San Francisco: Jossey-Bass.

Duff, R. S., Rowe, D. S., & Anderson, F. P. (1973). Patient care and student learning in a pediatric clinic. *Pediatrics, 50*, 839–846.

Dunn-Greier, B. J., McGarth, P. J., Rourke, B. P., Latter, J., & D'Astous, F. (1986). Adolescent chronic pain: The ability to cope. *Pain, 26*, 23–32.

DuRant, R. H., Rome, E. S., Rich, M., Allred, E., Emans, S. J., & Woods, E. R. (1997). Tobacco and alcohol use behaviors portrayed in music videos: A content analysis. *American Journal of Public Health, 87*, 1131–1135.

DuRant, R. H., Sanders, J. M., Jay, S., & Levinson, R. (1990). Adolescent contraceptive risk-taking behavior: A social psychological model of female's use of and compliance with birth control. In A. R. Stiffman & R. A. Feldman (Eds.), *Contraceptive use, pregnancy, and parenting* (pp. 87–106). London: Jessica Kingsley.

Edwards, L. N., & Grossman, M. (1978). *Children's health and the family.* Working Paper No. 256. Washington, DC: National Bureau of Economic Research.

———(1979). *Income and race differences in children's health.* Working Paper No. 308. Washington, DC: National Bureau of Economic Research.

Egbuonu, L., & Starfield, B. (1982). Child health and social status. *Pediatrics, 50,* 550–557.

Eiser, C. (1989). Children's concepts of illness: Towards an alternative to the "stage" approach. *Psychology and Health, 3,* 93–101.

Elder, J. P., Broyles, S. L., McKenzie, T. L., & Sallis, J. F. (1998). Direct home observations of the promoting of physical activity in sedentary and active Mexican- and Anglo-American children. *Journal of Developmental and Behavioral Pediatrics, 19,* 26–30.

Elinson, J., Henshaw, S., & Cohen, S. (1976). Responses by a low-income population to a multiphasic screening program: A sociological analysis. *Preventive Medicine, 5,* 414–424.

Ellison, R. C., Capper, A. L., Goldberg, R. J., Witschi, J. C., & Stare, F. J. (1989). The environmental component: Changing school food service to promote cardiovascular health. *Health Education Quarterly, 16,* 285–297.

Engel, G. L. (1977). The need for a new medical model: A challenge for biomedicine. *Science, 196,* 129–136.

Ennett, S. T., Bauman, K. E., Pemberton, M., & Foshee, V. A. (2001). Medication in a family-directed program for prevention of adolescent tobacco and alcohol use. *Preventive Medicine: An International Journal Devoted to Practice and Theory, 33,* 333–346.

Epstein, L. H., Paluch, R. A., Gordy, C. C., & Dorn, J. (2000). Decreasing sedentary behaviors in treating pediatric obesity. *Archives of Pediatrics and Adolescent Medicine, 154,* 220–226.

Farnya, E. L., & Morales, E. (2000). Self-efficacy and HIV-related risk behaviors among multiethnic adolescents. *Cultural Diversity and Ethnic Minority Psychology, 6,* 42–56.

Fassler, D., McQueen, K., Duncan, P., & Copeland, L. (1990). Children's perceptions of AIDS. *Journal of the American Academy of Child and Adolescent Psychiatry, 29,* 459–462.

Fearnow, M., Chassin, L., Presson, C. C., & Sherman, S. J. (1998). Determinants of parental attempts to deter their children's cigarette smoking. *Journal of Applied Developmental Psychology, 19,* 453–468.

Feeney, J. A. (2000). Implications of attachment style for patterns of health and illness. *Child Care, Health and Development, 26*, 277–288.

Feeney, J. A., & Ryan, S. M. (1994). Attachment style and affect regulation: Relationships with health behavior and family experiences of illness in a student sample. *Health Psychology, 13*, 334–345.

Feldman, S. S., & Rosenthal, D. A. (2000). The effect of communication characteristics on family members' perceptions of parents as sex educators. *Journal of Research on Adolescence, 10*, 119–150.

Field, D. (1987). *Child and parent coviewing of television: Relationships to cognitive performance.* Unpublished doctoral dissertation, University of Massachusetts, Amherst.

Fiese, B. H., & Sameroff, A. J. (1989). Family context in pediatric psychology: A transactional perspective. *Journal of Pediatric Psychology, 14*, 293–314.

Forehand, R., & Kotchick, B. A. (1996). Cultural diversity: A wake-up call for parent training. *Behavior Therapy, 27*, 187–206.

Forgays, D. K. (1992). Type A behavior and parenting stress in mothers with young children. *Current Psychology: Research & Reviews, 11*, 3–19.

Fors, S. W., Owen, S., Hall, N. D., McLaughlin, J., & Levinson, R. (1980). Evaluation of a diffusion strategy for school-based hypertension education. *Health Education Quarterly, 16*, 255–261.

Fothergill, K., & Ballard, E. (1998). The school-linked health center: A promising model of community-based care for adolescents. *Journal of Adolescent Health, 23*, 29–38.

Fowler, M. G., Simpson, G. A., & Schoendorf, K. C. (1993). Families on the move and children's health care. *Pediatrics, 91*, 934–940.

Fox, G. L., & Inazu, J. K. (1980). Patterns and outcomes of mother–daughter communication about sexuality. *Journal of Social Issues, 36*, 7–29.

Fraley, M. C., Nelson, E. C., Wolf, A. W., & Lozoff, B. (1991). Early genital naming. *Journal of Developmental and Behavioral Pediatrics, 12*, 301–304.

Frazer, J. G. (1959). *The golden bough: A study in magic and religion* (abridged; T. H. Gaster, Ed.). New York: Macmillan (original work published 1890).

Freedman, R. J. (1984). Reflections on beauty as it relates to health in adolescent females. *Women's Health, 9*, 29–45.

Friedman, M. A., & Brownell, K. D. (1995). Psychological correlates of obesity: Moving to the next research generation. *Psychological Bulletin, 117*, 3–20.

Frydman, M. (1999). Television, aggressiveness, and violence. *International Journal of Adolescent Medicine and Health, 11*, 335–344.

Furusho, J., Yamaguchi, K., Ikura, Y., Kogure, T., Suzuki, M., Konishi, S., Simizu, G., Nakayama, Y., Itoh, K., & Sakamoto, Y. (1998). Patient background of the Pokemon phenomenon: Questionnaire studies in multiple pediatric clinics. *Acta Paediatrica Japonica*, *40*, 550–554.

Gable, S., & Lutz, S. (2000). Household, parent, and child contributions to childhood obesity. *Family Relations: Interdisciplinary Journal of Applied Family Studies*, *49*, 293–300.

Gagnon, C., Vitaro, F., & Tremblay, R. E. (1992). Parent–teacher agreement on kindergartners' behavior problems. *Journal of Child Psychology and Psychiatry and Allied Disciplines*, *33*, 1255–1261.

Galst, J. P. (1980). Television food commercials and pronutritional public service announcements as determinants of young children's snack choice. *Child Development*, *51*, 935–938.

Garralda, M. E. (2000). The links between somatisation in children and in adults. In P. Reder & M. McClure (Eds.), *Family matters: Interfaces between child and adult mental health* (pp. 122–134). London: Rutledge.

Garrettson, L. K., Bush, J. P., Gates, R. S., & French, A. (1990). Physical change, time of day, and child characteristics as factors in poison injury. *Veterinary and Human Toxicology*, *32*, 139–141.

Garvey, C., & Berndt, R. (1977). Organization of pretend play. *Catalog of Selected Documents in Psychology*, *7*, 107.

Gault, A. R. (1990). Mexican immigrant parents and the education of their handicapped children: Factors that influence parent involvement. *Dissertation Abstracts International*, *50*(n7-A): 1865–1866.

Geasler, M. J., Dannison, L. L., & Edlund, C. J. (1995). Sexuality education of young children. *Family Relations*, *44*, 184–188.

Gellert, E. (1962). Children's conceptions of the content and functions of the human body. *Genetic Psychology Monographs*, *65*, 293–405.

Gerbner, G., Gross, L., Morgan, M., & Signorielli, N. (1980). The "mainstreaming" of America: Violence profile No. 9. *Journal of Communication*, *30*, 10–29.

Gerbner, G., Gross, L., Morgan, M., & Signorielli, N. (1981). *Aging with television commercials: Images on television commercials and dramatic programming, 1977–1979*. Unpublished manuscript, University of Pennsylvania, The Annenberg School of Communication, Philadelphia.

Gerbner, G., Gross, L., Signorielli, N., Morgan, M., & Jackson-Beeck, M. (1979). The demonstration of power: Violence Profile No. 10. *Journal of Communication*, *29*, 177–195.

Gissler, M., Jarvelink, M. R., Louhiala, P., & Hemminki, E. (1999). Boys have more health problems in childhood than girls: Follow-up of the 1987 Finnish birth cohort. *Acta Paediatrica*, *88*, 310–314.

Glascoe, F. P. (1999). Using parents' concerns to detect and address developmental and behavioral problems. *Journal of the Society of Pediatric Nurses, 4*, 24–35.

Gochman, D. S. (1987). *Youngsters' health cognitions: Cross-sectional and longitudinal analyses.* Louisville, KY: Health Behavior Systems.

Gochman, D. S. (1988a). Assessing children's health concepts. In P. Karoly (Ed.), *Handbook of child health assessment: Biopsychosocial perspectives* (pp. 332–356). New York: Wiley.

Gochman, D. S. (1988b). Health behavior: Plural perspectives. In D. S. Gochman (Ed.), *Health behavior: Emerging research perspectives* (pp. 3–12). New York: Plenum Press.

Gochman, D. S. (1997). Family health cognitions. In D. S. Gochman (ed.), *Handbook of health behavior research 1: Personal and social determinants* (pp. 207–221). New York: Plenum.

Godin, G., & Shephard, R. J. (1986). Psychosocial factors influencing intentions to exercise of young students from grades 7 to 9. *Research Quarterly for Exercise and Sport, 57*, 501–508.

Goldman, S. L., & Owen, M. T. (1994). The impact of parental trait anxiety on the utilization of health care services in infancy: A prospective study. *Journal of Pediatric Psychology, 19*, 369–381.

Gomez, C. A., & Marin, V. O. B. (1996). Gender, culture, and power: Barriers to HIV-prevention strategies for women. *The Journal of Sex Research, 33*, 3558–3662.

Gonzalez, J. C., Routh, D. K., Saab, P. G., Armstrong, F., Shifman, L., Guerra, E., & Fawcett, N. (1989). Effects of parent presence on children's reactions to injections: Behavioral, physiological, and subjective aspects. *Journal of Pediatric Psychology, 14*, 449–462.

Gorn, G. J., & Greenberg, M. E. (1982). Behavioral evidence of the effects of televised food messages on children. *Journal of Consumer Research, 9*, 200–205.

Gossler, J. L. (1980). *The study of the non-prescription vitamin giving behaviors of mothers of preschool and school-aged children.* Unpublished master's thesis, University of Oregon, Portland.

Gottman, J. M., & Katz, L. F. (1989). Effects of marital discord on young children's peer interaction and health. *Developmental Psychology, 25*, 373–381.

Gould, M. S., & Shaffer, D. (1989). The impact of suicide in television movies: Evidence of imitation. In R. F. W. Diekstra & R. Maris (Eds.), *Suicide and its prevention: The role of attitude and imitation* (pp. 331–340). Leiden, the Netherlands: E. J. Brill.

Graham, L., & Hamdan, L. (1987). *Youth trends: Capturing the $200 billion youth market.* New York: St. Martin's Press.

Gralinski, J. H., & Kopp, C. B. (1993). Everyday rules for behavior: Mothers' requests to young children. *Developmental Psychology, 29,* 573–584.

Greenberg, B. S., Linsangan, R., Soderman, A., Heeter, C., Lin, C., & Stanley, C. (1987). *Project CAST: Adolescents and their exposure to television and movie sex.* East Lansing: Communication Technology Laboratory, Michigan State University.

Greene, K., Rubin, D. L., Hale, J. L., & Walters, L. H. (1996). The utility of understanding adolescent egocentrism in designing health promotion messages. *Health Communication, 8,* 131–152.

Greenfield, P. M. (1984). *Mind and media: The effects of television, video games, and computers.* Cambridge, MA: Harvard University Press.

Greenfield, P. M., & Beagles-Roos, J. (1988). Television vs. radio: The cognitive impact on different socioeconomic and ethnic groups. *Journal of Communication, 38,* 71–92.

Greeson, L. E., & Williams, R. A. (1986). Social implications of music videos for youth: An analysis of the content and effects of MTV. *Youth and Society, 18,* 177–189.

Gross, A. M., Stern, R. M., Levin, R. B., Dale, J., & Wojnilower, D. A. (1983). The effect of mother–child separation on the behavior of children experiencing a diagnostic medical procedure. *Journal of Consulting and Clinical Psychology, 51,* 783–785.

Grube, J. W., & Wallack, L. (1994). Television beer advertising and drinking knowledge, beliefs, and intentions among schoolchildren. *American Journal of Public Health, 84,* 254–259.

Grundy, S. M. (2000). Early detection of high cholesterol levels in young adults. *Journal of the American Medical Association, 284,* 36–57.

Grusec, J. E., Goodnow, J. J., & Kuczynski, L. (2000). New directions in analyses of parenting contributions to children's acquisition of values. *Child Development, 71,* 205–211.

Grych, J. H., & Fincham, F. D. (1990). Marital conflict and children's adjustment: A cognitive-contextual framework. *Psychological Bulletin, 108,* 267–290.

Gunter, B., & McAleer, J. L. (1990). *Children and television: The one-eyed monster?* London: Routledge.

Gunzberg, R., Balague, F., Nordin, M., Szpalski, M., Duyck, D., Bull, D., & Melot, C. (1999). Low back pain in a population of school children. *European Spine Journal, 8,* 439–443.

Guske, S. J. (1980). *Factors determining the usage of infant car seats by mothers in the Kaiser Permanente Medical Program.* Unpublished master's thesis, University of Oregon, Portland.

Hacker, K., & Wessel, G. L. (1998). School-based health centers and school nurses: Cementing the collaboration. *Journal of School Health, 68,* 409–414.

Haefner, H., & Schmidtke, A. (1989). Increase of suicide due to imitation of fictional suicide on television. In B. Cooper & T. Helgason (Eds.), *Epidemiology and the prevention of mental disorders* (pp. 338–347). Florence, KY: Taylor & Francis/Routledge.

Halfon, N., Newacheck, P. W., Hughes, D., & Brindis, C. (1998). Community health monitoring: Taking the pulse of America's children. *Maternal and Child Health Journal, 2,* 95–109.

Hamburg, B. A., & Inoff, G. E. (1982). Relationships between behavioral factors and diabetic control in children and adolescents: A camp study. *Psychosomatic Medicine, 44,* 321–339.

Hammond, K. M., Wyllie, A., & Casswell, S. (1999). The extent and nature of televised food advertising to New Zealand children and adolescents. *Australian and New Zealand Journal of Public Health, 23,* 49–55.

Hanley, A. J., Harris, S. B., Gittlesohn, J., Wolever, T. M., Saksvig, B., & Zinman, B. (2000). Overweight among children and adolescents in a Native Canadian community: Prevalence and associated factors. *American Journal of Clinical Nutrition, 71,* 693–700.

Hanson, M. J., Lynch, E. W., & Wayman, K. I. (1990). Honoring the cultural diversity of families when gathering data. *Topics on Early Childhood Education, 10,* 112–131.

Harkness, S., & Keefer, C. H. (2000). Contributions of cross-cultural psychology to research and interventions in education and health. *Journal of Cross-Cultural Psychology, 31,* 92–109.

Harrison, K. (2000a). Television viewing, fat stereotyping, body shape standards, and eating disorder symptomatology in grade school children. *Communication Research, 27,* 617–640.

(2000b). The body electric: Thin-ideal media and eating disorders in adolescence. *Journal of Communication, 50,* 119–143.

Hartup, W. W. (1979). The social worlds of childhood. *American Psychologist, 8,* 76–79.

(1996). The company they keep: Friendships and their developmental significance. Society for Research in Child Development biennial meetings: Presidential address (1995, Indianapolis, IN). *Child Development, 67,* 1–13.

Hartup, W. W., & Stevens, N. (1999). Friendships and adaptation across the life span. *Current Directions in Psychological Science, 34,* 944–950.

Hatcher, J., Powers, L., & Richtsmeier, A. (1993). Parental anxiety and response to symptoms of minor illness in infants. *Journal of Pediatric Psychology, 18,* 397–408.

Hayes, C. (1987). Determinants of adolescent sexual behavior and decision making. In C. Hayes (Ed.), *Risking the future: Adolescent sexuality, pregnancy and childbearing* (Vol. 1, pp. 95–122). Washington, DC: National Academy Press.

Heck, K., & Parker, J. (1999). Family structure, socioeconomic status, and access to health care for children. *Abstract Book: Association for Health Services Research, 16,* 400.

Hei, T. K., & Gold, V. (1990, February). *Cholesterol levels of children who watch different amounts of television.* Paper presented at the annual meeting of the American Heart Association, Dallas.

Henggeler, S. W., Cohen, R., Edwards, J. J., & Summerville, M. B. (1991). Family stress as a link in the association between television viewing and achievement. *Child Study Journal, 21,* 1–10.

Hepburn, E. H. (1983). A three-level model of parent–daughter communication about sexual topics. *Adolescence, 18,* 523–534.

Hergenrather, J. R., & Rabinowitz, M. (1991). Age-related differences in the organization of children's knowledge of illness. *Developmental Psychology, 27,* 952–959.

Hernandez, B., Gortmacher, S. L., Colditz, G. A., Peterson, K. E., Laird, N. M., & Parra-Cabrera, S. (1999). Association of obesity with physical activity, television programs and other forms of video viewing among children in Mexico City. *International Journal of Obesity and Related Metabolic Disorders, 23,* 845–854.

Hertzman, C. (1999). The biological embedding of early experience and its effects on health in adulthood. *Annals of the New York Academy of Science, 896,* 85–95.

Hibbard, J. H., & Pope, C. R. (1993). The quality of social roles as predictors of morbidity and mortality. *Social Science and Medicine, 36,* 217–225.

Hodson, D. S., & Wampler, K. (1988). Social class and parental involvement in the sex education of children. *Journal of Sex Education and Therapy, 14,* 13–17.

Holland, P., Berney, L., Blane, D., Smith, G. D., Gunnell, D. J., & Montgomery, S. M. (2000). Life course accumulation of disadvantage: Childhood health and hazard exposure during adulthood. *Social Science and Medicine, 50,* 1285–1295.

Hooven, C., Gottman, J. M., & Katz, L. F. (1995). Parental meta-emotion structure predicts family and child outcomes. *Cognition and Emotion, 9,* 229–264.

Hotopf, M., Mayou, R., Wadsworth, M., & Wessely, S. (1999). Childhood risk factors for adults with medically unexplained symptoms: Results from a national birth cohort study. *American Journal of Psychiatry, 156,* 1796–1800.

Howard, M., & McCabe, J. A. (1992). An information and skills approach for younger teens: Postponing Sexual Involvement program. In B. C. Miller & J. J. Card (Eds.), *Preventing adolescent pregnancy: Model programs and evaluations* (pp. 83–109). Thousand Oaks, CA: Sage.

Howell-Koren, P., & Tinsley, B. J. (1990). The relationships among maternal health beliefs, pediatrician–mother communication, and maternal satisfaction with well-infant care. *Health Communication, 2,* 233–253.

Huesmann, L. R., Eron, L. D., Lefkowitz, M. M., & Walder, L. O. (1984). Stability of aggression over time and generations. *Developmental Psychology, 20,* 1120–1134.

Hupkens, C. L., Knibbe, R. A., Van Otterloo, A. H., & Drop, M. J. (1998). Class differences in the food rules mothers impose on their children: A cross-national study. *Social Science and Medicine, 47,* 1331–1339.

Huston, A. C., Donnerstein, E., Fairchild, H., Feshbach, N. D., Katz, P. A., Murray, J. P., Rubinstein, E. A., Wilcox, B. L., & Zuckerman, D. (1992). *Big world, small screen: The role of television in American society.* Lincoln: University of Nebraska Press.

Huston, A. C., & Wright, J. C. (1996). Television and socialization of young children. In T. M. MacBeth (Ed.), *Tuning into young viewers: Social science perspectives on television* (pp. 37–60). Thousand Oaks, CA: Sage.

  (1998). Mass media and children's development. In W. Damon (Gen. Ed.), I. E. Sigel, & K. A. Renninger (Vol. Eds.), *Handbook of child psychology* (Vol. 4, 4th ed., pp. 999–1058). New York: Wiley.

Hutchinson, K. M., & Cooney, T. M. (1998). Patterns of parent–teen sexual risk communication: Implications for intervention. *Family Relations: Interdisciplinary Journal of Applied Family Studies, 47,* 185–194.

Iannotti, R. J., & Bush, P. J. (1992). The development of autonomy in children's health behavior. In E. J. Susman, L. V. Feagans, & W. J. Ray (Eds.), *Emotion, cognition, health, and development in children and adolescents* (pp. 53–74). Hillsdale, NJ: Erlbaum.

Icard, L. D., Schilling, R. F., & El-Bassel, N. (1995). Reducing HIV infection among African Americans by targeting the African American family. *Social Work Research, 19,* 153–163.

Institute for Mental Health Initiatives. (1996). *Effects of television on children's mental health.* Washington, DC: Dunham Press.

Institute of Medicine. (1997). *The hidden epidemic: Confronting sexually transmitted diseases.* T. R. Eng & W. T. Butler (Eds.). Washington, DC: National Academy Press.

Jaccard, J., Dittus, P. J., & Gordon, V. V. (1998). Parent–adolescent congruence in reports of adolescents' sexual behavior and in communication about sexual behavior. *Child Development, 69,* 247–261.

(2000). Parent–teen communication about premarital sex: Factors associated with the extent of communication. *Journal of Adolescent Research, 15,* 187–208.

Jackson, R. W., Treiber, F. A., Turner, J. R., Davis, H., & Strong, W. B. (1999). Effects of race, sex, and socioeconomic status upon cardiovascular stress responsivity and recovery in youth. *International Journal of Psychotherapy, 31,* 111–119.

Jambor, E. (2001). Media involvement and the idea of beauty. In J. J. Robert-McComb (Ed.), *Eating disorders in women and children: Prevention, stress management, and treatment* (pp. 179–183). Boca Raton, FL: CRC Press.

Jeffrey, D. B., McClerran, R. W., & Fox, D. T. (1982). The development of children's eating habits: The role of television commercials. *Health Education Quarterly, 9,* 78–93.

Jessor, R. (1992). Risk behavior in adolescence: A psychosocial framework for understanding and action. *Developmental Review, 12,* 374–390.

Johnson, C., Birch, L. L., & McPhee, L. (1991). Conditioned preferences: Young children prefer flavors associated with high dietary fat. *Physiology and Behavior, 50,* 1245–1251.

Jones, E. F., Forrest, J. D., & Henshaw, S. K. (1988). Unintended pregnancy, contraceptive practice and family planning services in developed countries. *Family Planning Perspectives, 20,* 53–67.

Juanillo, N. K., Jr., & Scherer, C. W. (1991, July). *Patterns of family communication and health lifestyle.* Paper presented at the annual conference of the International Communication Association, Chicago.

Julian, T. W., McKenry, P. C., & McKelvey, M. W. (1991). Mediators of relationship stress between middle-aged fathers and their adolescent children. *Journal of Genetic Psychology, 152,* 381–386.

Kahlbaugh, P., Lefkowitz, E. S., Valdez, P., & Sigman, M. (1997). The affective nature of mother–adolescent communication concerning sexuality and conflict. *Journal of Research on Adolescence, 7,* 221–239.

Kalafat, J., & Illback, R. J. (1998). A qualitative evaluation of school-based family resource and youth service centers. *American Journal of Community Psychology, 26,* 573–604.

Kandel, D. B., Wu, P., & Davies, M. (1994). Maternal smoking during pregnancy and smoking by adolescent daughters. *American Journal of Public Health, 84,* 1407–1413.

Kasteleijn-Nolst Trenite, D. G., daSilva, A. M., Ricci, S., Binnie, C. D., Rubboli, G., Tassinari, C. A., & Segers, J. P. (1999). Video-game epilepsy: A European study. *Epilepsia, 40,* 70–74.

Katz, L. F., & Gottman, J. M. (1994). Patterns of marital interaction and children's emotional development. In R. D. Parke & S. G. Kellam

(Eds.), *Exploring family relationships with other social contexts* (pp. 49–74). Hillsdale, NJ: Erlbaum.

Kaufman, L. (1980). Prime time nutrition. *Journal of Communication, 30,* 37–46.

Kaune, W. T., Miller, M. C., Linet, M. S., Hatch, E. E., Kleinerman, R. A., Wacholder, S., Mohr, A. H., Tarone, R. E., & Haines, C. (2000). Children's exposure to magnetic fields produced by U.S. television sets used for viewing programs and playing video games. *Bioelectromagnetics, 21,* 214–227.

Kegeles, S., & Lund, A. K. (1982). Adolescents' health beliefs and acceptance of a novel preventive dental activity: Replication and extension. *Health Education Quarterly, 9,* 192–198.

Kenrick, D. T., & Gutierres, S. E. (1980). Contrast effects and judgements of physical attractiveness: When beauty becomes a social problem. *Journal of Personality and Social Psychology, 38,* 131–140.

Kiecolt-Glaser, J. K., & Glaser, R. (1995). Psychoneuroimmunology and health consequences: Data and shared mechanisms. *Psychosomatic Medicine, 57,* 269–274.

(2001). Stress and immunity: Age enhances the risks. *Current Directions in Psychological Science, 10,* 18–21.

Kiecolt-Glaser, J. K., & Newton, T. L. (2001). Marriage and health: His and hers. *Psychological Bulletin, 127,* 472–503.

Killen, J. D., Robinson, T. N., Telch, M. J., Saylor, K. E., Maron, D. S., Rich, T., & Bryson, S. (1989). The Stanford Adolescent Heart Health Program. *Health Education Quarterly, 16,* 263–283.

King, B. M., & Lorusso, J. (1997). Discussions in the home about sex: Different recollections by parents and children. *Journal of Sex and Marital Therapy, 23,* 52–60.

Kister, M. C., & Patterson, C. J. (1980). Children's conceptions of the causes of illness: Understanding of contagion and use of immanent justice. *Child Development, 51,* 839–846.

Klein, M., & Gordon, S. (1992). Sex education. In E. C. Walker & M. C. Roberts (Eds.), *Handbook of clinical child psychology* (2nd ed., pp. 933–949). New York: Wiley.

Klostermann, B. K., Perry, C. S., & Britto, M. T. (2000). Quality improvement in a school health program. Result of a process evaluation. *Evaluation and the Health Professions, 23,* 91–106.

Kobayashi, M., Takayama, H., Mihara, B., & Sugishita, M. (1999). Partial seizure with aphasic speech arrest caused by watching a popular animated TV program. *Epilepsia, 40,* 652–654.

Koblinsky, S., & Atkinson, J. (1982). Parental plans for children's sex education. *Family Relations, 31,* 29–35.

Kolody, B., & Sallis, J. F. (1995). A prospective study of ponderosity, body image, self-concept, and psychological variables in children. *Journal of Behavioral and Developmental Pediatrics, 16,* 1–5.

Kotchick, B. A., Shaffer, A., & Forehand, R. (2001). Adolescent sexual risk behavior: A multi-system perspective. *Clinical Psychology Review, 21,* 493–519.

Kramer, L., & Gottman, J. M. (1992). Becoming a sibling: "With a little help from my friends." *Developmental Psychology, 28,* 685–699.

Krauss, B. J. (1997). HIV education for teens and preteens in a high-seroprevalence inner-city neighborhood. *Families in Society, 78,* 579–591.

Krauss, B. J., Godfrey, C., Yee, D., Goldsamt, L., Tiffany, J., & Almeyda, L. (2000). *Saving our children from a silent epidemic: The PATH Program for parents and preadolescents.* Unpublished manuscript.

Kubey, R. W. (1986). Television use in everyday life: Coping with unstructured time. *Journal of Communication, 36,* 108–123.

Kubey, R. W., & Csikszentmihalyi, M. (1990). *Television and the quality of life: How viewing shapes everyday experience.* Hillsdale, NJ: Erlbaum.

Kunkel, D., Cope, K. M., Farinola, W. J. M., Biely, E., Rollin, E., & Donnerstein, E. (1999). *Sex on TV: Content and context.* Menlo Park, CA: Henry J. Kaiser Foundation.

Ladd, G. W., & LeSieur, K. D. (1995). Parents and children's peer relationships. In M. H. Bornstein (Ed.), *Handbook of parenting,* Vol. 4: *Applied and practical parenting* (pp. 377–409). Mahwah, NJ: Erlbaum.

LaGreca, A. M., Prinstein, M. J., & Fetter, M. D. (2001). Adolescent peer crowd affiliation: Linkages with health-risk behaviors and close friendships. *Journal of Pediatric Psychology, 26,* 131–143.

Landrine, H., Klonoff, E. A., Campbell, R., & Reina-Patton, A. (2000). Sociocultural variables in youth access to tobacco: Replication 5 years later. *Preventive Medicine: An International Journal Devoted to Practice and Theory, 30,* 433–437.

Larson, S. G. (1991). Television's mixed messages: Sexual content on *All My Children. Communication Quarterly, 39,* 156–163.

Lau, R. R., Hartman, K. A., & Ware, J. E. (1986). Health as a value: Methodological and theoretical considerations. *Health Psychology, 5,* 25–43.

Lau, R. R., & Klepper, S. (1988). The development of illness orientations in children aged 6 through 12. *Journal of Health and Social Behavior, 29,* 149–168.

Lau, R. R., Quadrel, M. J., & Hartman, K. A. (1990). Development and change of young adults' preventive health beliefs and behavior: Influence from parents and peers. *Journal of Health and Social Behavior, 31,* 240–250.

Lees, N. B., & Tinsley, B. J. (1998). Patterns of parental socialization of the preventive care of young Mexican origin children. *Journal of Applied Developmental Psychology, 19*, 503–525.

Lees, N. B., & Tinsley, B. J. (2000). Maternal socialization of children's preventive health behavior: The role of maternal affect and teaching strategies. *Merrill-Palmer Quarterly, 46*, 652–696.

Lefkowitz, E. S., Kahlbaugh, P. E., & Sigman, M. (1996). Turn-taking in mother–adolescent conversations about sexuality and conflict. *Journal of Youth and Adolescence, 25*, 307–321.

Leftwich, M. J. T., & Collins, F. L. (1994). Parental smoking, depression, and child development: Persistent and unanswered questions. *Journal of Pediatric Psychology, 19*, 557–569.

Leland, N. L., & Barth, R. P. (1993). Characteristics of adolescents who have attempted to avoid HIV and who have communicated with parents about sex. *Journal of Adolescent Research, 8*, 58–76.

Levenson, P. M., Copeland, D. R., Morrow, J. R., Pfefferbaum, B., and Silberberg, Y. (1983). Disparities in disease-related perceptions of adolescent cancer patients and their parents. *Journal of Pediatric Psychology, 8*, 33–35.

Levin, D. E. (1998). Food advertising on British children's television: A content analysis and experimental study with nine-year-olds. *International Journal of Obesity and Related Metabolic Disorders, 22*, 206–214.

LeVine, R. A. (1974). *Culture and personality: Contemporary readings.* Chicago: Aldine.

Leviton, L. C., Valdiserri, R. O., Lyter, D. W., & Callahan, C. M. (1990). Preventing HIV infection in gay and bisexual men: Experimental evaluation of attitude change from two risk reduction interventions. *HIV Education and Prevention, 2*, 95–108.

Lewis, C. E., & Lewis, M. A. (1974). The impact of television commercials on health-related beliefs and behavior of children. *Pediatrics, 53*, 431–435.

Lewis, C. E., and Lewis, M. A. (1982). Children's health-related decision making. *Health Education Quarterly, 9*, 225–237.

Liebert, R. M., & Sprafkin, J. (1988). *The early window – Effects of television on children and youth* (3rd ed.). New York: Pergamon Press.

Lightfoot, J., & Bines, W. (2000). Working to keep school children healthy: The complementary roles of school staff and school nurses. *Journal of Public Health Medicine, 22*, 74–80.

Lindquist, C. H., Reynolds, K. D., & Goran, M. I. (1999). Sociocultural determinants of physical activity among children. *Preventive Medicine, 129*, 305–312.

Livingston, R., Witt, A., & Smith, G. R. (1995). Families who somatize. *Journal of Developmental and Behavioral Pediatrics, 16*, 42–46.

Loveland-Cherry, C. J., Leech, S., Laetz, V. B., & Dielman, T. E. (1996). Correlates of alcohol use and misuse in fourth grade children: Psychosocial, peer, parental and family factors. *Health Education Quarterly*, *23*, 497–511.

Lowry, D. T., & Towles, D. E. (1989). Soap opera portrayals of sex, contraception, and sexually transmitted diseases. *Journal of Communication*, *39*, 76–83.

Luepker, R. V., Perry, C. L., Murray, D. M., & Mullis, R. (1988). Hypertension prevention through nutrition education in youth: A school-based program involving parents. *Health Psychology*, *7*, 233–245.

Lukoff, I. F (1980). Toward a sociology of drug use. In D. J. Lettieri, M. Sayers, & H. W. Pearson (Eds.), *Theories on drug abuse: Selected contemporary perspectives* (NIDA Research Monograph 30). Rockville, MD: National Institute on Drug Abuse.

MacKinnon, C. E., Lamb, M. E., Belsky, J., & Baum, C. (1990). An affective-cognitive model of mother–child aggression. *Development & Psychopathology*, *2*, 1–13.

Maiman, L. A., Becker, M. H., and Katlic, A. W. (1985). How mothers treat their children's physical symptoms. *Journal of Community Health*, *10*, 136–155.

Maiman, L. A., Becker, M. H., and Katlic, A. W. (1986). Correlates of mothers' use of medications for their children. *Social Science and Medicine*, *22*, 41–51.

Marcoux, M., Sallis, J. F., McKenzie, T. L., & Marshall, S. (1999). Process evaluation of a physical activity self-management program for children: SPARK. *Psychology and Health*, *14*, 659–677.

Main, M., Kaplan, N., & Cassidy, J. (1985). Security in infancy, childhood, and adulthood: A move to the level of representation. *Monographs of the Society for Research in Child Development*, *50*, 66–104.

Margolis, P. A., Keyes, L. L., Greenberg, R. A., Bauman, K. E., & LaVange, L. M. (1997). Urinary cotinine and parent history (questionnaire) as indicators of passive smoking and predictors of lower respiratory illness in infants. *Pediatric Pulmonology*, *23*, 417–423.

Markman, E. M. (1989). *Categorization and naming in children.* Cambridge, MA: MIT Press.

Matthews, S., Manor, O., & Power, C. (1999). Social inequalities in health: Are there gender differences? *Social Science and Medicine*, *48*, 49–60.

McElreath, L. H., & Roberts, M. C. (1992). Perceptions of acquired immune deficiency syndrome by children and their parents. *Journal of Pediatric Psychology*, *17*, 477–492.

McGillicuddy-DeLisi, A. V. (1992). Parents' beliefs and children's personal-social development. In I. E. Sigel & A. V. McGillicuddy-DeLisi (Eds.), *Parental belief systems: The psychological consequences for children* (2nd ed., pp. 115–142). Hillsdale, NJ: Erlbaum.

McKenzie, T. L., Nader, P. R., Strikmiller, P. K., & Yang, M. (1996). School physical education: Effect of the child and adolescent trial for cardiovascular health. *Preventive Medicine: An International Journal Devoted to Practice and Theory, 25*, 423–431.

Mechanic, D. (1965). Perception of parental responses to illness: A research note. *Journal of Health and Human Behavior, 6*, 253–257.

Mechanic, D. (1979). Correlates of physican utilization: Why do major multivariate studies of physician utilization find trivial psychosocial and organizational effects? *Journal of Health and Social Behavior, 20*, 389–396.

Mechanic, D. (1980). The experience and reporting of common physical complaints. *Journal of Health and Social Behavior, 21*, 146–155.

Melamed, B. G. (1998). Preparation for medical procedures. In R. T. Ammerman & J. V. Campos (Eds.), *Handbook of pediatric psychology, Vol. 2: Disease, injury, and illness* (pp. 16–30). Needham Heights, MA: Allyn & Bacon.

Mellanby, A. R., Rees, J. B., Tripp, J. H. (2000). Peer-led and adult-led school health education: A critical review of available comparative research. *Health Education Research, 15*, 533–545.

Meschke, L. L., Zweig, J. M., Barber, B. L., & Eccles, J. S. (2000). Demographic, biological, psychological, and social predictors of the timing of first intercourse. *Journal of Research on Adolescence, 10*, 315–338.

Messaris, P., & Sarett, C. (1981). On the consequences of television-related parent–child interaction. *Human Communication Research, 7*, 226–244.

Meyers, C. (1992). Hmong children and their families. *Journal of Occupational Therapy, 46*, 955.

Midford, R., & McBride, N. (2001). Alcohol education in schools. In N. Heather & T. J. Peters (Eds.), *International handbook of alcohol dependence and problems* (pp. 785–804). New York: Wiley.

Miller, K. S., Forehand, R., & Kotchick, B. A. (1999). Adolescent sexual behavior in two ethnic minority samples: The role of family variables. *Journal of Marriage and the Family, 61*, 85–98.

Miller, K. S., Forehand, R., & Kotchick, B. A. (2000). Adolescent sexual behavior in two ethnic minority groups: A multisystem perspective. *Adolescence, 35*, 313–333.

Miller, K. S., Kotchick, B., Dorsey, S., Forehand, R., & Ham, A. (2001). Family communication about sex: What are parents saying and are their adolescents listening? *Family Planning Perspectives, 30*, 218–222.

Miller, K., Levin, M. L., Whitaker, D. J., & Xu, X. (1998). Patterns of condom use among adolescents: The impact of maternal–adolescent communication. *American Journal of Public Health, 88*, 1542–1544.

Miller, P. H. (2000). *Theories of developmental psychology* (4th ed.). New York: Freeman.

Milovsky, J. R., Pekowsky, B., & Stipp, H. (1975–1976). TV drug advertising and proprietary and illicit drug use among boys. *Public Opinion Quarterly, 39*, 457–481.

Minuchin, P. (1985). Families and individual development: Provocations from the field of family therapy. *Child Development, 56*, 289–302.

Mishara, B. L. (1999). Conceptions of death and suicide in children ages 6–12 and their implications for suicide prevention. *Suicide and Life-Threatening Behavior, 29*, 105–118.

Montgomery, K. (2000). Youth and digital media: A policy research agenda. *Journal of Adolescent Health, 27*, 61–68.

Moore, L. L., Lombardi, D. A., White, M. J., Campbell, J. L., Oliveria, S. A., & Ellison, R. C. (1991). Influence of parents' physical activity levels on activity levels of young children. *The Journal of Pediatrics, 118*, 215–219.

Moran, J. R., & Corley, M. D. (1991). Sources of sexual information and sexual attitudes and behaviors of Anglo and Hispanic adolescent males. *Adolescence, 26*, 857–864.

Morgan, M. (1988). Cultivation analysis. In E. Barnouw (Ed.), *International encyclopedia of communication* (Vol. 1, pp. 430–433). New York: Oxford University Press.

Morse, A. E., Hyde, J. J., Newberger, E. H., & Reed, R. B. (1977). Environmental correlates of pediatric social illness: Preventive implications of an advocacy approach. *American Journal of Public Health, 67*, 612–615.

Mukai, T., Crago, M., & Shisslak, C. M. (1994). Eating attitudes and weight preoccupation among female high school students in Japan. *Journal of Child Psychology and Psychiatry and Allied Disciplines, 35*, 677–688.

Murray, M., Kiryluk, S., & Swan, A. V. (1985). Relation between parents' and children's smoking behaviour and attitudes. *Journal of Epidemiology and Community Health, 39*, 169–174.

Murry, V. M. (1996). An ecological analysis of coital timing among middle-class African American adolescent females. *Journal of Adolescent Research, 11*, 261–279.

Nader, P. R., Sellers, D. E., Johnson, C. C., & Perry, C. L. (1996). The effect of adult participation in a school-based family intervention to improve children's diet and physical activity: The child and adolescent trial for cardiovascular health. *Preventive Medicine: An International Journal Devoted to Practice and Theory, 25*, 455–464.

Nagy, M. (1951). Children's ideas on the origins of illness. *Health Education Journal, 9*, 6–12.

(1953). The representation of "germs" by children. *Journal of Genetic Psychology, 83*, 227–240.

Natapoff, J. N. (1978). Children's views of health: A developmental study. *American Journal of Public Health, 68*, 995–1000.

National Center for Children in Poverty. (1995). *Five million children: A statistical profile of our poorest young citizens.* New York: Columbia University School of Public Health.

Nelson, I. (1986). *Event knowledge: Structure and function in development.* Hillsdale, NJ: Erlbaum.

Nemeroff, C. J. (1995). Magical thinking about illness virulence: Conceptions of germs from "safe" versus "dangerous" others. *Health Psychology, 14*, 147–151.

Neuhauser, C., Amsterdam, B., Hines, P., & Steward, M. (1978). Children's concepts of healing: Cognitive development and locus of control factors. *American Journal of Orthopsychiatry, 48*, 335–341.

Newcomb, A. F., Bukowski, W. M., & Pattee, L. (1993). Children's peer relations: A meta-analytic review of popular, rejected, neglected, controversial and average sociometric status. *Psychological Bulletin, 113*, 99–128.

Newcomer, S. F., & Udry, J. R. (1985). Oral sex in an adolescent population. *Archives of Sexual Behavior, 14*, 41–46.

Nicholls, J. G., & Miller, A. I. (1983). The differentiation of the concepts of difficulty and ability. *Child Development, 54*, 951–959.

Nolin, M. J., & Petersen, K. K. (1992). Gender differences in parent–child communication about sexuality: An exploratory study. *Journal of Adolescent Research, 7*, 59–79.

Noll, R. B., Zucker, R. A., & Greenberg, G. S. (1990). Identification of alcohol by smell among preschoolers: Evidence for early socialization about drugs occurring in the home. *Child Development, 61*, 1520–1527.

Noller, P., & Callan, V. J. (1990). Adolescents' perceptions of the nature of their communication with parents. *Journal of Youth and Adolescence, 19*, 349–362.

Normandeau, S., Kalnins, I., Jutras, S., & Hanigan, D. (1998). A description of 5- to 12-year-old children's conception of health within the context of their daily life. *Psychology and Health, 13*, 883–896.

O'Donnell, L., Stueve, A., Doval, A. S., & Duran, R. (1999). The effectiveness of the Reach for Health community youth service learning program in reducing early and unprotected sex among urban middle school students. *American Journal of Public Health, 89*, 176–181.

Oetting, E. R., & Beauvais, F. (1987). Common elements in youth drug abuse: Peer clusters and other psychosocial factors. *Journal of Drug Issues, 17*, 133–151.

O'Leary, A. (1990). Stress, emotion, and human immune function. *Psychological Bulletin, 108,* 363–382.

Olvera-Ezzell, N., Power, T. G., & Cousins, J. H. (1990). Maternal socialization of children's eating habits: Strategies used by obese Mexican-American mothers. *Child Development, 61,* 395–400.

Olvera-Ezzell, N., Power, T. G., & Cousins, J. H. (1990). Maternal socialization of children's eating habits: Strategies used by obese Mexican-American mothers. *Child Development, 61,* 395–400.

Owens, J., Maxim, R., McGuinn, M., Nobile, C., Msall, M., & Alario, A. (1999). Television viewing habits and sleep disturbance in school children. *Pediatrics, 104,* 27.

Parcel, G. S., Bruhn, J. G., & Murray, J. L. (1983). Preschool Health Education Program (PHEP): Analysis of educational and behavioral outcome. *Health Education Quarterly, 10,* 149–172.

Parcel, G. S., Bruhn, J. G., & Murray, J. L. (1984). Effects of a health education curriculum on the smoking intentions of preschool children. *Health Education Quarterly, 11,* 49–56.

Parcel, G. S., & Meyer, M. P. (1978). Development of an instrument to measure children's health locus of control. *Health Education Monographs, 6,* 149–159.

Parcel, G. S., Simons-Morton, B., O'Hara, N. M., Baranowski, T., & Wilson, B. (1989). School promotion of health, diet, and physical activity: Impact on learning outcomes and self-reported behavior. *Health Education Quarterly, 16,* 181–189.

Parke, R. D. (2000). Father involvement: A developmental psychological perspective. *Marriage and Family Review, 29,* 43–58.

Parke, R. D., & Bhavnagri, N. P. (1989). Parents as managers of children's peer relationships. In D. Belle (Ed.), *Children's social networks and social supports* (pp. 241–259). New York: Wiley.

Parker, J. G., Rubin, K. H., Price, J. M., & DeRosier, M. E. (1995). Peer relationships, child development and adjustment: A developmental psychopathology perspective. In D. Cicchetti & D. Cohen (Eds.), *Developmental psychopathology,* Vol. 2: *Risk disorder and adaptation* (pp. 96–161). New York: Wiley.

Parmelee, A. H., Jr. (1986). Children's illnesses: Their beneficial effects on behavioral development. *Child Development, 57,* 1–10.

Parmelee, A. H., Jr. (1992). Wellness, illness, health, and disease concepts. In E. J. Susman & L. V. Feagans (Eds.), *Emotion, cognition, health, and development in children and adolescents* (pp. 155–164). Hillsdale, NJ: Erlbaum.

Parmelee, A. H., Jr. (1997). Illness and the development of social competence. *Journal of Developmental and Behavioral Pediatrics, 18,* 120–124.

Patterson, G. R., Capaldi, D., & Bank, L. (1991). An early starter model for predicting delinquency. In D. J. Pepler & K. H. Rubin (Eds.), *The development and treatment of childhood aggression* (pp. 139–168). Hillsdale, NJ: Erlbaum.

Patterson, G. R., DeBaryshe, B. D., & Ramsey, E. (1989). A developmental perspective on antisocial behavior. *American Psychologist, 44*, 329–335.

Pebley, A., Hurtado, E., & Goldman, N. (1999). Beliefs about children's illness. *Journal of Biosocial Science, 31*, 195–219.

Perrin, E. C., & Gerrity, P. S. (1981). There's a demon in your belly: Children's understanding of illness. *Pediatrics, 67*, 841–849.

Perrino, T., Gonzalez-Soldevilla, A., Pantin, H., & Szapoczick, J. (2000). The role of families in adolescent HIV prevention. *Clinical Child and Family Psychology Review, 3*, 81–96.

Perry, C. L., Sellers, D. E., Johnson, C., & Pedersen, S. (1997). The Child and Adolescent Trial for Cardiovascular Health (CATCH): Intervention, implementation, and feasibility for elementary schools in the United States. *Health Education and Behavior, 24*, 716–735.

Perusse, L., Tremblay, A., LeBlanc, C., & Bouchard, C. (1989). Genetic and environmental influences on level of habitual physical activity and exercise participation. *American Journal of Epidemiology, 129*, 1012–1022.

Peterson, C., & Seligman, M. E. P. (1987). Explanatory style and illness. *Journal of Personality, 55*, 238–265.

Peterson, L., Bartelstone, J., Kern, T., & Gillies, R. (1995). Parents' socialization of children's injury prevention: Description and some initial parameters. *Child Development, 66*, 224–235.

Peterson, L., Farmer, J., & Kashani, J. H. (1990). Parental injury prevention endeavors: A function of health beliefs? *Health Psychology, 9*, 177–191.

Peterson, P. E., Jeffrey, D. G., Bridgwater, C. A., & Dawson, B. (1984). How pronutrition television programming affects children's dietary habits. *Developmental Psychology, 20*, 55–63.

Phillips, D. P., Carstensen, L. L., & Paight, D. J. (1989). Effects of mass media news stories on suicide, with new evidence on the role of story content. In C. R. Pfeffer (Ed.), *Suicide among youth: Perspectives on risk and prevention* (pp. 106–116). Washington, DC: American Psychiatric Press.

Pillado, O., Romo, L. F., & Sigman, M. (2000, March). *The influence of Latino mother characteristics on the content of dating and sexuality talks with their teenagers.* Paper presented at the meetings of the Society for Research on Adolescence, Chicago.

Potts, R., Doppler, M., & Hernandez, M. (1994). Effects of television content on physical risk-taking in children. *Journal of Experimental Child Psychology, 58*, 321–331.

Potts, R., Runyan, D., Zerger, A., & Marchetti, K. (1996). A content analysis of safety behaviors of television characters: Implications for children's safety and injury. *Journal of Pediatric Psychology, 21*, 517–528.

Potts, R., & Swisher, L. (1998). Effects of televised safety models on children's risk taking and hazard identification. *Journal of Pediatric Psychology, 23*, 157–163.

Prabhu, N. P., Duffy, L. C, & Stapleton, F. B. (1996). Content analysis of prime-time television medical news. A pediatric perspective. *Archives of Pediatrics and Adolescent Medicine, 150*, 46–49.

Pratkanis, A. R., Breckler, S. J., & Greenwald, A. G. (Eds.). (1989). *Attitude structure and function*. Hillsdale, NJ: Erlbaum.

Pratt, L. (1973). Child-rearing methods and children's health behaviors. *Journal of Health and Social Behavior, 14*, 61–69.

Princeton Survey Research Associates, Inc. (1994). *Children's Health Index*. Emmaus, PA: *Prevention* magazine.

Radius, S. M., Dillman, T. E., Becker, M. H., Rosenstock, I. M., & Horvath, W. J. (1980). Adolescent perspectives on health and illness. *Adolescence, 15*, 375–384.

Raffaelli, M., Bogenschneider, K., & Flood, M. F. (1998). Parent–teen communication about sexual topics. *Journal of Family Issues, 19*, 315–333.

Ramey, C. T., MacPhee, D., & Yeates, K. (1982). Preventing developmental retardation: A systems theory approach. In L. Bond & J. Joffe (Eds.), *Primary prevention of psychopathology* (pp. 279–299). Hanover, NH: University Press of New England.

Ranelli, P. L., Bartsch, K., & London, K. (2000). Pharmacists' perceptions of children and families as medicine consumers. *Psychology and Health, 15*, 829–840.

Rashkis, S. R. (1965). Child's understanding of health. *American Medical Association Archives of General Psychiatry, 12*, 10–17.

Ratner, H. H., & Stettner, L. J. (1991). Thinking and feeling: Putting Humpty Dumpty together again. *Merrill-Palmer Quarterly, 37*, 1–26.

Reading, R., Langford, I. H., Haynes, R., & Lovett, A. (1999). Accidents to preschool children: Comparing family and neighbourhood risk factors. *Social Science and Medicine, 48*, 321–330.

Reisch, L. M., Tinsley, B. J., & Phillips, G. M. (1994, June). *Intergenerational transmission of explanatory style for health events*. Paper presented at the meetings of the International Society for the Study of Behavioural Development, Amsterdam.

Reiss, D. (1989). Families and their paradigms: An ecological approach to understanding the family in its social world. In C. N. Ramsey Jr. (Ed.), *Family systems in medicine* (pp. 119–134). New York: Guilford Press.

Resnick, M. D. (1990). Study group report on the impact of televised drinking and alcohol advertising on youth. *Journal of Adolescent Health Care, 11,* 25–30.

Reyes, M. B., Routh, D. K., Jean-Gilles, M. M. & Sanfilippo, M. D. (1991). Ethnic differences in parenting children in fearful situations. *Journal of Pediatric Psychology, 16,* 717–726.

Ricciuti, H. N. (1980). Developmental consequences of malnutrition in early childhood. In M. Lewis & L. Rosenblum (Eds.), *The uncommon child: The genesis of development* (Vol. 3, pp. 129–139). New York: Plenum.

Richter, K. P., Harris, K. J., Paine-Andrews, A., & Fawcett, S. B. (2000). Measuring the health environment for physical activity and nutrition among youth: A review of the literature and applications for community initiatives. *Preventive Medicine: An International Journal Devoted to Practice and Theory, 31,* S98–S111.

Richtsmeier, A. J., & Hatcher, J. W. (1994). Parental anxiety and minor illness. *Journal of Developmental and Behavioral Pediatrics, 15,* 14–19.

Rickard, K. (1988). The occurrence of maladaptive health-related behaviors and teacher-rated conduct problems in children of chronic low back pain patients. *Journal of Behavioral Medicine, 11,* 107–116.

Roberts, D. F. (2000). Media and youth: Access, exposure, and privatization. *Journal of Adolescent Health, 27,* 8–14.

Roberts, E., Kline, D., & Gagnon, J. (1978). *Family life and sexual learning: A study of the role of parents in the sexual learning of children.* Cambridge, MA: Population Education.

Robinson, J. O., Alverez, J. H., & Dodge, K. A. (1990). Life events and family history in children with recurrent abdominal pain. *Journal of Psychosomatic Research, 34,* 171–181.

Robinson, J. P. (1972). Television's impact on everyday life: Some cross-national evidence. In E. A. Rubinstein, G. A. Comstock, & J. P. Murray (Eds.), *Television and social behavior,* Vol. 4: *Television in day-to-day life: Patterns of use* (pp. 143–156). Washington, DC: Government Printing Office.

Rogers, K. D., & Reese, G. (1965). Health studies – presumably normal high school students: II. Absence from school. *American Journal of Diseases of Children, 109,* 9–27.

Roghmann, K. J., Hecht, P. K., & Haggerty, R. J. (1973). Family coping with everyday illness: Self-reports from a household survey. *Journal of Comparative Family Studies, 4,* 49–62.

Rogoff, B. (1997). Evaluating development in the process of participation: Theory, methods, and practice building on each other. In E. Amsel & K. A. Renninger (Eds.), *Change and development: Issues of theory, method, and application* (pp. 265–285). Mahwah, NJ: Erlbaum.

Rokeach, M. (1974). Change and stability in American value systems, 1968–1971. *Public Opinion Quarterly, 38,* 222–238.

Romelsjo, A. (1987). Decline in alcohol-related problems in Sweden greatest among young people. *British Journal of Addiction, 82,* 1111–1124.

Rosenstock, I. M., & Kirscht, J. P. (1980). Why people seek health care. In G. L. Stone, F. Cohen, & N. E. Adler (Eds.), *Health psychology – A handbook* (pp. 161–188). San Francisco: Jossey-Bass.

Rosenthal, D., & Feldman, S. S. (1999). The importance of importance: Parent–adolescent communication about sexuality. *Journal of Adolescence, 22,* 835–852.

Rossiter, J. R., & Robertson, T. S. (1980). Children's dispositions toward proprietary drugs and the role of television drug advertising. *Public Opinion Quarterly, 44,* 316–329.

Rozin, P., Fallon, A., & Augustoni-Ziskind, M. (1985). The child's conception of food: The development of contamination sensitivity to "disgusting" substances. *Developmental Psychology, 21,* 1075–1079.

Rozin, P., Markwith, M., & McCauley, C. (1994). The nature of aversion to indirect contacts with other persons: AIDS aversion as a composite of aversion to strangers, infection, moral taint, and misfortune. *Journal of Abnormal Psychology, 103,* 495–504.

Rubovits, D. S., & Wolynn, T. H. (1999). Children's illness cognitions: What mothers think. *Clinical Pediatrics, 38,* 99–105.

Rushforth, H. (1999). Communicating with hospitalised children: Review and application of research pertaining to children's understanding of health and illness. *Journal of Child Psychology and Psychiatry and Allied Disciplines, 40,* 683–691.

Rutter, M. (2000). Resilience reconsidered: Conceptual considerations, empirical findings, and policy implications. In J. P. Shonkoff & S. J. Meisels (Eds.), *Handbook of early childhood intervention* (2nd ed., pp. 651–682). New York: Cambridge University Press.

Sallis, J. F., Patrick, K., Frank, E., & Pratt, M. (2000). Interventions in health care settings to promote healthful eating and physical activity in children and adolescents. *Preventive Medicine, 31,* 5112–5120.

Sallis, J. F., Alcaraz, J. E., McKenzie, T. L., Hovell, M. F., Kolody, B., & Nader, P. R. (1992). Parental behavior in relation to physical activity and fitness in 9-year-old children. *American Journal of Diseases of Children, 146,* 1383–1388.

Sallis, J. F., Patterson, T. L., Buono, M. J., Atkins, C. J., & Nader, P. R. (1988). Aggregation of physical activity habits in Mexican-American and Anglo families. *Journal of Behavioral Medicine, 11*, 31–41.

Sameroff, A. J. (1982). Development and the dialectic: The need for a systems approach. In W. A. Collins (Ed.), *Minnesota Symposium on Child Psychology* (Vol. 15, pp. 179–203). Hillsdale, NJ: Erlbaum.

Sameroff, A. J. (1989). General systems and the regulation of development. In M. Gunnar & E. Thelen (Eds.), *Systems and development* (pp. 219–236). Hillsdale, NJ: Erlbaum.

Sameroff, A. J. (1998). Environmental risk factors in infancy. *Pediatrics, 102*, 1287–1292.

Sameroff, A. J., & Chandler, M. J. (1975). Reproductive risk and the continuum of caretaking casualty. In F. Horowitz (Ed.), *Review of child development research* (Vol. 4, pp. 293–321). Chicago: University of Chicago Press.

Sameroff, A. J., Seifer, R., Zax, M., & Barocas, R. (1987). Early indicators of developmental risk: Rochester longitudinal study. *Schizophrenia Bulletin, 13*, 383–394.

Sandler, I. N., Miller, P., Short, J., & Wolchik, S. A. (1989). Social support as a protective factor for children in stress. In D. Belle (Ed.), *Children's support networks and social supports* (pp. 297–307). New York: Wiley.

Sanger, M. S., Sandler, H. K., & Perrin, E. C. (1988). Concepts of illness and perceptions of control in healthy children and children with chronic illnesses. *Journal of Developmental and Behavioral Pediatrics, 9*, 252–256.

Santelli, J., DiClemente, R., Miller, K., & Kirby, D. (1999). Sexually transmitted diseases, unintended pregnancy, and adolescent health promotion. In M. Fisher, L. Juszczak, & L. Klerman (Eds.), *Adolescent medicine: Prevention issues in adolescent health care* (Vol. 10, pp. 87–108). San Francisco: Jossey-Bass.

Sarafino, E. P. (1990). *Health psychology: Biopsychosocial interactions*. New York: Wiley.

Sarason, I. G., Sarason, B. R., & Pierce, G. R. (1992). The contexts of social support. In H. O. F. Veiel & U. Baumann (Eds.), *The meaning and measurement of social support* (pp. 143–154). Washington, DC: Hemisphere.

Schaefer, E. S. (1979). Professional paradigms in child and family health programs. *American Journal of Public Health, 69*, 849–850.

Scheer, S. D., Borden, L. M., & Donnermeyer, J. F. (2000). The relationship between family factors and adolescent substance use in rural, suburban, and urban settings. *Journal of Child and Family Studies, 9*, 105–115.

Schetky, D. (1985). Children and handguns: A public health concern. *American Journal of Diseases of Children, 139*, 229–231.

Schilling, R. F., El-Bassel, N., Leeper, M. A., & Freeman, L. Gilbert, L., & Schinke, S. P. (1991). Acceptance of the female condom by Latin- and African-American women. *American Journal of Public Health, 81*, 1345–1346.

Schor, E. S., Starfield, B., Stidley, C., & Hankin, J. (1987). Family health: Utilization and effects of family membership. *Medical Care, 25*, 616–626.

Scott-Jones, D., & Turner, C. (1990). The impact of adolescent childbearing on educational attainment and income of black females. *Youth and Society, 22*, 35–53.

Shakato, R., Edwards, L., & Grossman, M. (1980). *An exploration of the dynamic relationship between health and cognitive development in adolescence.* Working Paper No. 454. Washington, DC: National Bureau of Economic Research.

Shaw, E. G., & Routh, D. K. (1982). Effect of mother presence on children's reaction to aversive procedures. *Journal of Pediatric Psychology, 7*, 33–42.

Sherman, B. L., & Dominick, J. R. (1986). Violence and sex in music video: TV and rock'n' roll. *Journal of Communication, 36*, 79–93.

Shrier, L. A., Harris, S. K., Sternberg, M. & Beardslee, W. R. (2001). Associations of depression, self-esteem, and substance use with sexual risk among adolescents. *Preventive Medicine, 33*, 179–189.

Siegal, M. (1991). *Knowing children: Experiments in conversation and cognition.* Hillsdale, NJ: Erlbaum.

Siegal, M., & Peterson, C. C. (1999). Becoming mindful of biology and health: An introduction. In M. S. Siegal & C. C. Peterson (Eds.), *Children's understanding of biology and health* (pp. 1–19). New York: Cambridge University Press.

Sigel, I. E., & Dorval, B. (2000). Groundwork for a holistic view of the ontogenesis of representation. In N. Budwig & I. C. Uzgiris (Eds.), *Communication: An arena of development* (pp. 169–193). Stamford, CT: Ablex.

Sigelman, C. K., Derenowski, E. B., Mullaney, H. A., & Siders, A. T. (1993). Parents' contributions to knowledge and attitudes regarding HIV. *Journal of Pediatric Psychology, 18*, 221–235.

Sigelman, C. K., Leach, D. B., Mack, K. L., & Bridges, L. J. (2000). Children's beliefs about long-term health effects of alcohol and cocaine use. *Journal of Pediatric Psychology, 25*, 557–566.

Sigman, M. (1995). Nutrition and child development: More food for thought. *Current Directions in Psychological Science, 4*, 52–55.

Signorielli, N., & Lears, M. (1992). Television and children's conceptions of nutrition: Unhealthy messages. *Health Communication, 4*, 245–257.

Silverstein, B., Peterson, B., & Perdue, L. (1986). Some correlates of the thin standard of bodily attractiveness for women. *International Journal of Eating Disorders, 5*, 907–916.

Simarski, J. W. (1998). The birds and bees: An analysis of advice given to parents through the popular press. *Adolescence, 33*, 33–45.

Simeonsson, R. J., Buckley, L., & Monson, L. (1979). Conceptions of illness causality in hospitalized children. *Journal of Pediatric Psychology, 4*, 77–84.

Simpkins, S. D., & Parke, R. D. (2001). The relations between parental friendships and children's friendships: Self-report and observational analysis. *Child Development, 72*, 569–582.

Singer, D. G., & Singer, J. L. (Eds.). (2000). *Handbook of children and the media*. Thousand Oaks, CA: Sage.

Singer, L., Arendt, R., Farkas, K., & Minnes, S. (1997). Relationship of prenatal cocaine exposure and maternal postpartum psychological distress to child developmental outcome. *Development and Psychopathology, 9*, 473–489.

Smetana, J. G. (1988). Adolescents' and parents' conceptions of parental authority. *Child Development, 59*, 321–335.

Smetana, J. G., Kochanska, G., & Chuang, S. (2000). Mothers' conceptions of everyday rules for young toddlers: A longitudinal investigation. *Merrill-Palmer Quarterly, 46*, 391–416.

Somers, C. L., & Paulson, S. E. (2000). Students' perceptions of parent–adolescent closeness and communication about sexuality: Relations with sexual knowledge, attitudes, and behaviors. *Journal of Adolescence, 23*, 629–644.

Spotts, J. V., & Shontz, F. C. (1984). Drugs and personality: Extraversion-introversion. *Journal of Clinical Psychology, 40*, 624–628.

Spruijt-Metz, D. (1999). *Adolescence, affect, and health*. Hove, East Sussix, UK: Psychology Press.

Sroufe, L. A., & Fleeson, J. (1986). Attachment and the construction of relationships. In W. W. Hartup & Z. Rubin (Eds.), *Relationships and development* (pp. 51–71). Hillsdale, NJ: Erlbaum.

St. Peters, M., Fitch, M., Huston, A. C., & Wright, J. C. (1991). Television and families: What do young children watch with their parents? *Child Development, 62*, 1409–1423.

Stamler, C., & Palmer, J. O. (1971). Dependency and repetitive visits to the nurse's office in elementary school children. *Nursing Research, 20*, 254–255.

Stein, J. A., & Newcomb, M. D. (1994). Children's internalizing and externalizing behaviors and maternal health problems. *Journal of Pediatric Psychology, 19*, 571–593.

Steinberg, L. D. (1986). Latchkey children and susceptibility to peer pressure: An ecological analysis. *Developmental Psychology*, *22*, 433–439.

Steinberg, L. D., Lamborn, S. D., Dornbusch, S. M., & Darling, N. (1992). Impact of parenting practices on adolescent achievement: Authoritative parenting, school involvement and encouragement to succeed. *Child Development*, *63*, 1266–1281.

Stephens, B. K., Barkey, M. E., & Hall, H. R. (1999). Techniques to comfort children during stressful procedures. *Advances in Mind-Body Medicine*, *15*, 49–60.

Steward, M. S., & Steward, D. S. (1981). Children's conceptions of medical procedures. In R. Bibace & M. Walsh (Eds.), *New directions for child development: Children's conceptions of health, illness, and bodily functions*, No. 14. San Francisco: Jossey-Bass.

Stone, E. J., Perry, C. L., & Luepker, R. V. (1989). Synthesis of cardiovascular behavioral research for youth health promotion. *Health Education Quarterly*, *16*, 155–169.

Stone, P. W., Teutsch, S., Chapman, R. H., Bell, C., Goldie, S. J., & Neumann, P. J. (2000). Cost-utility analyses of clinical preventive services: Published ratios, 1976–1997. *American Journal of Preventive Medicine*, *19*, 15–23.

Strasburger, V. C. (1989). Children, adolescents, and television 1989 – II. The role of the pediatrician. *Pediatrics*, *83*, 446–448.

Strasburger, V. C. (1990). Television and adolescents: Sex, drugs, rock 'n' roll. *Adolescent Medicine: State of the Art Review*, *1*, 161–194.

Strasburger, V. C. (1992). Children, adolescents, and television. *Pediatrics in Review*, *13*, 144–151.

Strasburger, V. C. (1995). *Adolescents and the media: Medical and psychological impact*. Thousand Oaks, CA: Sage.

Strasburger, V. C., & Donnerstein, E. (1999). Children, adolescents, and the media: Issues and solutions. *Pediatrics*, *103*, 129–139.

Strasburger, V. C., & Donnerstein, E. (2000). Children, adolescents, and the media in the 21st century. *Adolescent Medicine*, *11*, 51–68.

Strasburger, V. C., & Hendren, R. L. (1995). Rock music and music videos. *Pediatric Annals*, *24*, 97–103.

Strouse, J. S., Buerkel-Rothfuss, N., & Long, E. C. J. (1995). Gender and family as moderators of the relationship between music video exposure and adolescent sexual permissiveness. *Adolescence*, *30*, 505–521.

Sussman, S. (2001). School-based tobacco use prevention and cessation: Where are we going? *American Journal of Health Behavior*, *25*, 191–199.

Takada, H., Aso, K., Watanabe, K., Okumura, A., Negoro, T., & Ishikawa, T. (1999). Epileptic seizures induced by animated cartoon, "Pocket Monster." *Epilepsia*, *40*, 997–1002.

Tan, A. (1979). TV beauty ads and role expectations of adolescent female viewers. *Journalism Quarterly, 56*, 283–288.

Tanasecu, M., Ferris, A. M., Himmelgreen, D. A., Rodriguez, N., & Perez-Escamilla, R. (2000). Biobehavioral factors are associated with obesity in Puerto Rican children. *Journal of Nutrition, 130*, 1734–1742.

Taylor, S. E. (1999). *Health psychology* (4th ed.). New York: McGraw-Hill.

Thomasgard, M., & Metz, W. P. (1995). The vulnerable child syndrome revisited. *Journal of Developmental and Behavioral Pediatrics, 16*, 47–53.

Tinsley, B. J. (1992). Multiple influences on the acquisition and socialization of children's health attitudes and behavior: An integrative review. *Child Development, 63*, 1043–1069.

Tinsley, B. J. (1997). Maternal influences on children's health behavior. In D. S. Gochman (Ed.), *Handbook of health behavior research 1: Personal and social determinants* (pp. 223–240). New York: Plenum.

Tinsley, B. J., & Holtgrave, D. R. (1989). Parental health beliefs, utilization of childhood preventive health services and infant health. *Journal of Developmental and Behavioral Pediatrics, 10*, 236–241.

Tinsley, B. J., & Lees, N. B. (1995). Health promotion for parents. In M. H. Bornstein (Ed.), *Handbook of parenting*, Vol. 4: *Applied and practical parenting* (pp. 187–204). Mahwah, NJ: Erlbaum.

Tinsley, B. J., Markey, C. N., Ericksen, A. J., Kwasman, A., & Ortiz, R. V. (2002). Health promotion for parents. In M. H. Bornstein (Ed.), *Handbook of parenting* (Vol. 5, 2nd ed.). Mahwah, NJ: Erlbaum.

Tinsley, B. J., & Parke, R. D. (1984). The historical and contemporary relationship between developmental psychology and pediatrics: A review and empirical survey. In H. E. Fitzgerald, B. M. Lester, & M. W. Yogman (Eds.), *Theory and research in behavioral pediatrics* (pp. 2–30). New York: Plenum.

Tinsley, B. J., Trupin, S. R., Owens, L., & Boyum, L. A. (1993). The significance of women's pregnancy control beliefs for adherence to recommended prenatal health regimens and pregnancy outcomes. *Journal of Reproductive and Infant Psychology, 11*, 97–102.

Tobia, A., Wolfson, A., & Gallagher, K. (1995, April). *The influence of negative uncontrollable life events on sleep and waking behaviors in kindergartners.* Paper presented at the biennial meetings of the Society for Research on Child Development, Indianapolis.

Toyamo, N. (2000). "What are food and air like inside our bodies?": Children's thinking about digestion and respiration. *International Journal of Behavior and Development, 24*, 222–230.

Tremblay, R. E., Masse, B., Perron, D., LeBlanc, M., Schwartzman, A. E., & Ledingham, J. E. (1992). Early disruptive behavior, poor school achievement, delinquent behavior and delinquent personality: Longitudinal analysis. *Journal of Consulting and Clinical Psychology*, *60*, 64–72.

Unnikrishnan, N., & Bajpai, S. (1996). *The impact of television advertising on children*. Thousand Oaks, CA: Sage.

Valerio, M., Amodio, P., Dalzio, M., Vianello, A., & Zacchello, G. P. (1997). The use of television in 2- and 8-year-old children and the attitude of parents about such use. *Archives of Pediatrics and Adolescent Medicine*, *151*, 22–26.

Valsiner, J., & Lightfoot, C. (1987). Process structure of parent–child–environment relations and the prevention of children's injuries. *Journal of Social Issues*, *43*, 61–72.

Van Arsdell, W. R., Roghmann, K. J., & Nader, P. R. (1972). Visits to an elementary school nurse. *Journal of School Health*, *42*, 142–147.

Verbrugge, L. M. (1983). Multiple roles and physical health of men and women. *Journal of Health and Social Behavior*, *24*, 16–30.

Vignerova, J., Blaha, P., Kobzova, J., Krejcovsky, L., Paulova, M., & Riedlova, J. (2000). Results of a multifactor cardiovascular risk reduction program in the Czech Republic: The healthy Dubic Project. *Central European Journal of Public Health*, *1*, 21–23.

Vygotsky, L. S., Rieber, R. W., & Carton, A. S. (1987). *The collected works of L. S. Vygotsky*, Vol. 1: *Problems of general psychology*. New York: Plenum.

Walker, L. S., & Greene, J. W. (1987). Negative life events, psychosocial resources, and psychophysiological symptoms in adolescents. *Journal of Clinical Child Psychology*, *16*, 29–36.

Walker, L. S., & Zeman, J. L. (1992). Parental response to child illness behavior. *Journal of Pediatric Psychology*, *17*, 49–71.

Wallston, K. A., Wallston, B. S., Smith, S., & Dobbins, C. J. (1987). Perceived control and health. In M. Johnston & T. Marteau (Eds.), *Applications in health psychology* (pp. 5–25). New Brunswick, NJ: Transaction.

Walsh, M. E., & Bibace, R. (1991). Children's conceptions of HIV: A developmental analysis. *Journal of Pediatric Psychology*, *16*, 273–285.

Walter, H. J. (1989). Primary prevention of chronic disease among children: The school-based "know your body" intervention trials. *Health Education Quarterly*, *16*, 201–214.

Ward, L. M., & Rivadeneyra, R. (1999). Contributions of entertainment television to adolescents' sexual attitudes and expectations: The role of viewing amount versus view involvement. *Journal of Sex Research*, *36*, 237–249.

Warton, P. M., & Goodnow, J. J. (1991). The nature of responsibility: Children's understanding of "your job." *Child Development, 62,* 156–165.

Weeks, K., Levy, S. R., Gordon, A. K., & Handler, A. (1997). Does parental involvement make a difference? Impact of parent interactive activities on students in a school-based HIV prevention program. *HIV Education and Prevention, 9,* 90–106.

Weinberg, A. D., Carbonari, J. P., & Laufman, L. (1984). What high school students don't know about cardiovascular disease. *Journal of School Health, 54,* 112–117.

Weisenberg, M., Kegeles, S. S., & Lund, A. K. (1980). Children's health beliefs and acceptance of a dental preventive activity. *Journal of Health and Social Behavior, 21,* 59–74.

Weist, M. D. (2001). Toward a public mental health promotion and intervention system for youth. *Journal of School Health, 71,* 101–104.

Wertlieb, D., Hauser, S. T., & Jacobson, A. M. (1986). Adaptation to diabetes: Behavior symptoms and family context. *Journal of Pediatric Psychology, 11,* 463–479.

Whitaker, D. D., & Miller, K. (2000). Parent–adolescent discussions about sex and condoms: Impact on peer influences on sexual behavior. *Journal of Adolescent Research, 15,* 251–273.

White, J. L., Moffitt, T. E., Earls, F., Robins, L., & Silva, P. A. (1990). How early can we tell? Predictors of childhood conduct disorder and adolescent delinquency. *Criminology, 28,* 507–533.

Wiehl, L. G., & Tinsley, B. J. (1999). Maternal personality and health communication in the pediatric context. *Health Communication, 11,* 75–96.

Wilkinson, S. R. (1988). *The child's world of illness: The development of health and illness behaviour.* Cambridge: Cambridge University Press.

Williams, T. H., & Handford, A. G. (1986). Television and other leisure activities. In T. H. Williams (Ed.), *The impact of television: A natural experiment in three communities* (pp. 152–171). Orlando, FL: Academic Press.

Wilson, N., Quigley, R., & Mansoor, O. (1999). Food ads on TV: A health hazard for children? *Australian and New Zealand Journal of Public Health, 23,* 647–650.

Winston, F. K., Duyck Wolff, K., Jordan, A., & Bhatia, E. (2000). Actions without consequences: Injury-related messages in children's programs. *Archives of Pediatrics and Adolescent Medicine, 154,* 366–369.

Wolin, S. J., & Bennett, L. A. (1984). Family rituals. *Family Process, 23,* 401–420.

Wood, B. L., Klebba, K. B., & Miller, B. D. (2000). Evolving the biobehavioral family model: The fit of attachment. *Family Process, 39,* 319–344.

Woodring, B. C. (1998). Relationship of physical activity and television watching with body weight and level of fatness among children: Results from the Third National Health and Nutrition Examination Survey. *Journal of Child and Family Nursing, 1,* 78–79.

Wurtele, S. K. (1993). Enhancing children's sexual development through child sexual abuse prevention programs. *Journal of Sex Education and Therapy, 19,* 37–46.

Yamasaki, K. (1990). Parental child-rearing attitudes associated with Type A behaviors in children. *Psychological Reports, 67,* 235–239.

Yamasaki, K. (1995). Development of Type A characteristics as a personality. *Japanese Psychological Review, 38,* 1–24.

Yowell, C. (1997). Risks of communication: Early adolescent girls' conversations with mothers and friends about sexuality. *Journal of Early Adolescence, 17,* 172–196.

Zahn-Waxler, C., Radke-Yarrow, M., & King, R. A. (1979). Child rearing and children's prosocial initiations toward victims of distress. *Child Development, 50,* 319–330.

Zero Population Growth. (1993). *Stress and where children live.* Washington, DC: Author.

Zillman, D., & Vorderer, P. (Eds.). (2000). *Media entertainment: The psychology of its appeal.* Mahwah, NJ: Erlbaum.

Index